Ahisha Fergu

Stops

DIET ~~STARTS~~ MONDAY

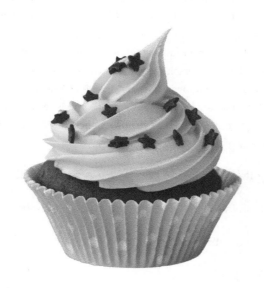

CONTENTS

DEDICATION

*For **Mum***

It took for me to lose you before I began to find myself.

You showed me how to be brave.

Always on my mind.

Forever in my heart.

Miss you always.

ACKNOWLEDGEMENTS

Firstly, a massive thank you to my wonderful husband Josh, who has put up with so much and been my back bone when I lost mine.

To my wonderful test readers, who were the first people to get their hands on this book. You all gave me courage to keep going, knowing this book could help millions of women like you finally start loving their bodies again and reach their goals.

To Danni, at Conscious Dreams Publishing who encouraged me from the very start. She believed in me before I believed in myself.

To my wonderful editors and proofreaders, Wendy and Anna Yorke, who added the polishing touches and made the structure of my book work for my readers.

And last but not least, to my Mum and Dad. You taught me to reach for the stars to achieve my full potential and to always follow my dreams.

THIS BOOK IS FOR YOU IF YOU...

- are fed up with feeling hungry all the time from dieting;
- are tired of feeling guilty every time you eat;
- are constantly blaming yourself for failing all the time;
- have tried it all before and simply want to know the secret to permanent weightloss;
- have been searching for the perfect way to lose weight without dieting; and
- are truly ready to lose weight and keep it off for good.

Enough is enough, forget everything else you have tried before, remember it isn't you, it's them!

You can have success by:
- following the simple truths in this book;
- without dieting;
- by forgetting all the rubbish you have been told before about eating less food; and
- without starving yourself or setting foot in a gym!

WHAT OTHER PEOPLE ARE SAYING
ABOUT THIS BOOK

"Last year, at a time like this I felt very low, blamed myself for not achieving the weight or eating lifestyle I desired. I was unhappy and didn't feel good enough. Initially, I thought it would be a long book with technical terms and phrases on nutrition and weightloss. I thought it was going to be the usual unrealistic goal oriented material. But this is one of the easiest to read books I have ever come across! I felt like Ahisha was speaking to me all along and was right there with me on a new journey, I can almost hear her voice. The diagrams are genius and the structure is great, makes it easy to grasp. This book is quite honest and factual. It focuses on what we don't hear a lot. This book empowered me to look after myself for myself and not for the image of society.

I learned from reading this book that my perspective of diet changed as I realised that I had to engage in a habit, which is a lifestyle and have a clear defined goal, finding ways to reward myself along the way. Now, I can enjoy the ride rather than blaming myself for the past; knowing that asking for help is okay."

Tabitha Kavoi, National Health Service

"I decided to read this book because I have dieted in so many different ways and they never work for long, but I need a permanent lifestyle change so that I can lose weight and keep it off forever. This book described my whole life inside and out, it made me laugh and at times, feel a little emotional. It was a very easy but informative read.

I learned that I need to love myself and my body even though its lumpy and bumpy! I don't have to go without food to be able to lose weight. I now realise diet is a bad word! It is a long-term lifestyle choice, not a faddy diet, which will help you in the long run and I don't need to feel guilty any more about eating."

Ruth Douglas, Nursery Manager

"Great easy read. I loved how I could relate to my past habits and some occasional ones I still have. Love the bit about when you are happy to write 10 things; great idea. I'm a huge foodie. Love the myth debunking and the questions to make us aware and think. Awesome read, wow. Thanks for letting me read it. Also, it gave me the kick up the backside I needed. I know what to do now. Felt like I took lots of nuggets from the book too. Highly recommended."

Stacey Humphris Blackley, Cake Baker

"As a professional dancer, I have always been very slim, fit and healthy. However; since the death of my mother 3 years ago, I have barely danced and it has really affected my weight. I was very keen to read this book and gain insights.

I love the way Ahisha writes, as if she is sitting right next to you talking directly to you, like a friend. I love the way she is not preachy, yet is clearly knowledgeable. I also really like how she busts several myths out the window. I really liked the diagrams that came with several sections. I also learned a lot about myself as an emotional eater from the various questions that were asked. This is not only a book about weightloss that reveals the truth about dieting and why it so often works against us, but *it is a book about self-discovery and raises awareness on so many levels about why we diet and why it doesn't work. I thoroughly enjoyed every aspect of it and learned so much. It was really interesting to learn about the visceral fat levels in people with the same waist circumference: that was a big surprise to me. How to detox effectively was a biggie for me and really important as I know how good I feel when I feel clean from the inside. I also learned how to set a goal and not beat myself up."*

Glynis Wozniak, Professional Performer

"We have been wanting to lose weight for a while and wondered if all the 'tailor made diets' were worthwhile or not. This book was easy to read and easy to understand. We learned that cutting down your food isn't always the best solution and you can still lose weight while eating your favourite things. We also discovered that you should still consume the amount of calories that you should have and not restrict and starve yourself."

Kerry Ann O'Conner, Student and Tracy O'Conner, Carer

"Reading this book felt like I was getting a talking to and I love that about it. I love that it's open to exploring the truth about ourselves and what we put into our bodies. It was a smooth read and I never felt anything was held back. I feel everything that is written is said for a reason – to aid us – I earnt that we should actually be doing the opposite to what we are told are the fundamentals to weightloss. I love that I learned more about the myths of dieting, but more importantly why they are myths. I love the fact that I feel like I have my own personal Health Coach in a book!"

Rio Gibbs, Magazine Owner

A WORD FROM THE AUTHOR

Hi! I wasn't sure how to start this book, to be honest. I had the word "Hi!" written for quite a while before I thought of something to say…and let's face it…I've still not said much have I?

I will begin by saying, thank you. Thank you for purchasing this book. More than anything I want to get this book out to help women like you who are sick and tired of dieting. Women who want to feel empowered by their food choices instead of guilty. Women who have tried it all, only to be frustrated that nothing works for long. Women who are at the end of their tether and want something simple to lose weight and finally keep it off for good. Believe me, I know it isn't easy to eat healthy and stay off the sugar and the booze. Yes, of course, we want to look sexy, but we want the wine too right? I know I am not alone when I say that! We want to have our cake and eat it.

Well, I am here to say that now we can do exactly that. It **is** possible to have it all. It is possible to lose weight without calorie counting and cutting meals and I am going to make one thing clear to start with. It is **not** your fault that up until now you have not succeeded. I repeat, it is **not** your fault! I will talk about this more in the first section of this book, but you need to know and accept that it isn't your fault before you can move forward. Stop blaming yourself for being 'fat' and stop blaming yourself for 'not having any willpower.' It simply isn't true and

15

the sooner you accept that the better. You are enough. You can do this. You have everything it takes within you to have the success you have been looking for. Throughout the sections of this book I will show you why it isn't your fault and I will show you the top reasons why you aren't losing weight and how you can overcome them.

However, I raise a warning here. I will be sharing cold hard facts and revealing secrets from the diet industry, which will challenge what you believe currently to be true. I will be challenging you to question your current beliefs and asking you to be open minded about learning a **new** truth. If you aren't ready for a new truth, put this book down slowly and back away because this book is not for you.

However, if you know you are **really** ready to hear the **real** truth and find out why you have failed at every weightloss attempt before…keep reading. If you are ready for a breakthrough and if you are ready to finally lose weight and keep it off without dieting, then let's get on with it!

See you on the other side. Health and happiness.

Ahisha x

INTRODUCTION:

Are You Ready To Give Up Dieting?

Did you know the word 'diet' is one of my least favourite words? I literally cannot stand it when I hear women say, "My diet starts again on Monday!" I cringe every time because I know exactly how it will end. It will be finished by Thursday and start again the following Monday. Sound familiar? This is why the book is entitled **Diet Stops Monday**, because it is time to stop the madness and get healthy for real this time, not simply until next Monday...

During the years the definition of the word 'diet' has become misplaced and women all over the world believe that to lose weight, they must exercise vigorously and go on a 'diet'. The way we understand and use the word 'diet' is totally misconstrued.

Celebrities and so called public 'role models' in the spotlight fuel this notion further to fatten their bank accounts by creating or endorsing these crazy fad diets and claiming the 'diet' is what makes them look so perfect!

In reality, most celebs are not doing these fad diets they talk about and promote. We have to remember that most of them have an entourage of people around them to help them look the way they do. It isn't the 'diet' they are endorsing that makes them look the way they do. They have personal trainers who come to their home each day to motivate them and they might have a personal chef and even a nutritionist on hand to educate them about food and cook for them. They have clothes tailored to fit them perfectly so they don't look lumpy or bumpy. They have airbrushing done in magazines or even worse, they might have surgery!

It isn't only the celebs who are offering false hope either. It is sadly also the 'professionals' sometimes too. I know of a nutrition colleague who developed a 2 month weightloss programme but wanted to get more clients to grow her business. What she decided to do was to announce to everyone that she was doing her own programme and would share her results at the end (to prove that it worked). Which in theory is a great idea.

However, she revealed to me that "life had got in the way" and she didn't end up completing her own program. However, rather than come clean and tell the world the truth, she decided to take laxatives and have colonic irrigations, to shed the weight fast towards the end of the 2 months, so she could 'prove' her great results. She then posted a picture of her start weight and finish weight for all to see. With no one knowing the truth, on the surface it certainly looked like her 2 month program had worked. Think about the Body Coach himself, Mr Joe Wicks, who admitted he had been living on junk food for many months.

Now, I can't say whether or not their programs work. Maybe they do. But what I can say clearly is that these programs aren't as simple or easy as they lead us to believe. Otherwise, they would have been able to stick to their **own** programs and achieve the results they have been promising us.

Weightloss isn't as easy as eating less food and counting calories. If it were, then everyone would have done it by now. There is a psychology and a science to weightloss, which simply isn't spoken about in public.

This only adds to those feelings of guilt and failure when we can't achieve those promised results for ourselves. For this reason, I have vowed to always have full transparency, which you will see in this book. I am not perfect and I refuse to offer any type of false hope because it isn't fair to anyone and quite frankly, you deserve better.

Us mere mortal regular women look at these celebs and so called professionals in the public eye and wonder why we aren't as perfect as them. We put ourselves down because we put these people up on a pedestal. But remember, the celebs have a team of professionals on hand for almost everything and what we see in the media isn't always what it may seem. We need to stop aspiring to have celeb bodies and comparing ourselves with them. What you think they have, they don't have, so you are looking for something that in reality doesn't exist. Aspiring to look like those celebs does nothing but set us up for disappointment and more dieting.

As for me, I have been through my own program and I'm currently working through my own emotional eating myself. It's not a quick fix and I continue to work on it all the time, which is why you won't see me displaying before and after photos. I am a work in progress and that is normal. In fact, we are all a work in progress. When you get to know me... you will also get to know how much I love cake! But at the same time my day to day life style is healthier than most...and more importantly you will never catch me going on a diet!

What is a 'diet' anyway?

I desperately want to clear up the way the word 'diet' is used in our day-to-day vocabulary. Understand the difference between 'your diet' and 'going on a diet'.

Going on a diet is something temporary and short-term and short-term 'diets' give short-term and temporary results.

ur diet is what you eat in general; your lifestyle, day-to-day, day in and day out. Your diet and day-to-day lifestyle is what will get you the permanent results you want without the constant cycles of going on a diet.

Examples of a faddy short term diet that you can go on are the liquid diet, the low fat diet, the cabbage soup diet, the Atkins diet, the calorie restriction diet, the water or juice fast...the next diet that will be released will probably be the AIR diet!

These short-term diets are simply not sustainable. It would be almost impossible to live on them day to day and make them your permanent every day diet. You would eventually burn out, get headaches and go down right crazy! Going on diets makes most women miserable and unhappy. Restricting your natural instinct to **eat real food** while dieting is also linked to bouts of binge eating or insane junk food binging too, which then makes us feel guilty. While there are a minority of people who succeed with these diet regimes, more than 80% of people who lose weight on diets gain it all back again and some, within 2 years or less. Also, did you know there is a massive financial disadvantage of short-term diets? Because these temporary diets give temporary results, people tend to try out a variety of diets in search of THE ONE that will work. As a result, the average amount of money women will end up spending on diets in their lifetime accumulates to a whopping £25,000! That's a deposit on a house! Imagine what else you could spend that money on if you gave up dieting! My goodness, you could go on a few cruises with that money! Given the choice would you spend the money on dieting or cruising? I know what my money is on!

The dangers of continuously dieting

Aside from the financial downside, let us also take a second to consider how dangerous some of these diets are for our bodies and overall health. Engaging in fad diets can ruin your metabolism. And I don't mean ruin it for a little while. You can wreck your metabolism FOR LIFE. This means that when you actually decide to give up 'dieting' and lose weight by permanently changing your lifestyle to something that is sustainable and healthy, your metabolism can be so screwed up that it will be even harder than necessary for you to lose weight later on. YIKES!

Even worse, extreme on and off dieting can also add stress and pressure on your body as well as your mind. Not only can dieting leave you feeling depressed and full of anxiety about your weight, it can also increase your chances of cancer, liver kidney and heart problems. Dr Atkins, creator of the famous Atkins diet, suffered cardiac arrests, heart disease and was a whopping 18 stone when he passed away only aged 72! Dieting is not healthy. It doesn't make us happy and leaves us feeling like failures. Think about it, on your last diet how did you feel when you 'fell off the wagon?' How did you feel when you couldn't say "No" to that slice of pizza? How do you feel when your friends ask the dreaded question, "How's the diet going?" or "I thought you were on a diet?" all the while knowing deep down you have failed that diet again. How many times have you said, "I'm starting again on Monday" or "Next time it will be different" and you get to Monday, or that next time comes around and you fail yet again? I know how I feel about that. I feel disheartened. I feel like I'm not good enough! I feel like nothing ever works for me. I feel like a failure. I feel downright embarrassed! This dieting nonsense does absolutely nothing for our self-esteem and it permanently effects our metabolism with all the start, stop, start, stop, merry go round malarky. My head is all a tizz simply thinking about dieting!

We have to really start to think about what we are doing to our bodies and our minds when we embark on these temporary diets over and over again.

Do you want to finally lose weight forever?
(And eat real food, not only lettuce leaves like a rabbit!)

The key to a successful 'diet' is to find a sustainable and permanent way to eat, which becomes your diet for **life** that you can live by **always**. It becomes your lifestyle and what you eat day to day permanently without you feeling deprived. Changing the DIET MINDSET will change your life and you will NEVER feel like it's a struggle again. Your life long diet shouldn't involve strict calorie, point or syn counting. It should not involve replacing more than one meal with a liquid and it should not include regular consumption of pre-packaged ready-made meals. This is not sustainable or healthy for your body in the long term.

Your everyday diet for weightloss and weight maintenance should be a mental and lifestyle change and should include a personal decision to be more educated on food, ingredients, label reading and understanding your body so you can make truly EDUCATED decisions about what you put into your body. Also, it shouldn't solely focus on fitting in to that dress or those skinny jeans or looking good on a beach. While this may be important to some people, this shouldn't be the sole purpose because it isn't sustainable and sooner or later you will slip back into old habits. Your everyday new and improved diet should be a step-by-step process to gradually changing your whole attitude towards the food you eat. It should make you feel ALIVE and excited about food!

This is an aspect that my team and I are dedicated to. When I say team, I mean my husband Josh and I. We have been nicknamed The Nutrition PAs by our clients because we are like the personal assistants for anything health and food related. We give every one of our client's key **knowledge** about food to create a healthier permanent diet and lifestyle for good. Our clients leave us with a newfound love of cooking and food in general. Most importantly, our clients leave us feeling GOOD about food. We help them create a lifestyle where they can actually eat REAL

FOOD and not sit around fighting cravings or starving themselves for a big event or holiday coming up. We look at NUTRIENTS, not calories and encourage them to eat real, good food. We are absolutely dedicated and committed to changing the dieting mindset and empowering women to take back control of their weight, their health and showing them how to LOVE food again without any guilt. I am so passionate about what we do that I decided to jot down my best-kept secrets for you to have and cherish forever within this book. For you to finally have success and see that the failings you have experienced before and which has lead you to the point of purchasing this book are NOT YOUR FAULT!

It is not your fault

Did you know, most weightloss companies don't actually want you to lose weight and keep it off? Yes, you read that right. That diet club you joined doesn't actually want you to succeed. Well, they do at first, but not forever. The biggest kept secret in the dieting industry is that weightloss companies and diet clubs only want you to lose weight initially, so you get what you want and you are a happy customer and go on your merry way. Left to your own devices however, the likelihood is you go back to normal, the weight creeps back on and you feel like a failure, but where do you turn? Back to another diet because it worked before, right? You get back in diet mode, lose weight, feel happy, go back to normal, put the weight on, feel like a failure, go back to the diet etc.

Have a look at my pretty diagram below. I am a visual person and I have dotted pictures for you to check out throughout this book. Does the diagram ring any bells for you?

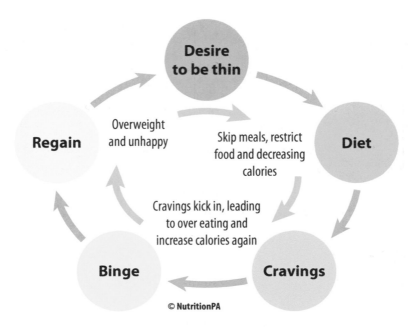

This is a fundamental flaw in nearly every diet system. Most diets you have tried before are almost impossible to keep up long term...as in for the rest of your life, because most of them rely on the basis that you need to remove food or calories for a short period of time. You cannot count every single calorie, weigh every meal and count every point or every syn for the rest of your life. You certainly will not last very long if you try to live on 1000 calories per day, permanently. Regular diets teach you to lose weight by eating less food, but when you go back to eating normally, the weight comes back so you have no choice but to go on ANOTHER diet.

It is time to rethink your diet mentality because put quite simply diets like that do not work. Everything you currently know about dieting and weightloss is a big fat lie and it is not your fault that it hasn't worked for you yet. You have been told that to lose weight you need to exercise more and eat less food...while it can work for some people yes, this doesn't work for most people. We have had many clients lose weight by eating MORE food than they were before and exercising moderately. Not by skipping meals and working out every day of the week, doing insane running and cardio. Eating less food and doing crazy work out regimes doesn't last long. You get tired, you get hungry, you get cravings and falling off the wagon is inevitable. Some of these diets are so extreme that it becomes so easy to fall off the dieting wagon. On that note, here is my biggest tip for not falling off the wagon. Are you ready for it? My biggest tip for how to not fall off the wagon is to not get on one in the first place! That's it! Simple, right? Press the buzzer, jump off at the next stop and let that diet wagon roll on by. You don't need it. Say your goodbyes. It's time to break up with dieting for good and the truth is; you deserve better. You would need super human willpower to stick to strict regimes for the rest of your life. Trust me. It is not you, it is them! It is an old cliché, but has never been truer than now. It is time to end that love hate relationship you have with food and dieting because it isn't working and in the end you start to blame yourself.

Failing at dieting and blaming yourself starts to grind your confidence down. You start to feel like you aren't good enough or like you are a failure. I have been there and know it all too well. You see all these before and after photos on the Internet and wonder why it's not working like that for you. Well, here is another secret. Many of those before and after photos are taken a month or so apart when they get their first initial result. If they did **another** photoshoot which showed the after the **after** photo, you would see that a year down the line, those people look exactly like they did in that very first before photo...or worse. The after the **after** photo is NEVER shown in public so when YOU fail, you believe it is **only** you who is failing and it is **your** fault. I met someone who shared with me that they have their face plastered across certain diet clubs flyers because they had amazing results some years ago. However, since that after photo was taken and his story was shared, he had regained all the weight he had initially lost and more! That **after** the after photo will never be shared and all people see is the previous success story leading you to think it MUST be you doing it wrong. But

I am here to say it is not your fault. Every other woman who is dieting, is like you and has the **after** the after photo which is kept private. A massive 80% of women dieting in the UK lose weight and put it all back on and more within 2 years. In fact, women in the UK will end up losing their entire body weight 9 TIMES in their lifetime. Oh and remember the other fun statistical fact about dieting? The one where you end up spending more than £25,000 on dieting? That is a lot of money. Think of how many holidays you could have had or that house you could have bought if only you weren't dieting all the time!

Again, don't blame yourself. These weightloss companies and diet clubs have great advertising. They are marketing masters. But let us be logical for a moment. If they all REALLY worked...there would be less and less people using them right...because they have all achieved success already. Think about it. If dieting truly was the miracle we have all been looking for, you wouldn't be here reading this book. You wouldn't feel like a failure because you would already have the body of your dreams. If dieting worked we wouldn't be in the situation we are today in Britain. According to the National Government statistics, in 2015 58% of women and 68% of men were overweight or obese. Obesity prevalence in 1993 was 15% and rose to a 27% in 2015. What is worse is that children are also now being affected. In 2015/16, more than 1 in 5 children in Reception, and more than 1 in 3 children in Year 6 were measured as obese or overweight. If all the traditional methods of dieting worked, none of that would be a problem would it? In fact, we would all have the body of our dreams...but we don't because dieting doesn't work and that isn't our fault. But **now** we can finally know the truth. Now you can become wise. Now you can have this knowledge. Let us do this right so you can finally have the success you deserve. Decide here and now to stop all the food counting and start loving your body enough to feed it the nutrients it needs. Accept that there is no quick fix and this will take some time. After all, you have spent your entire life doing things a certain way and created bad habits, which you will have to break and that will take time and effort. But I know you aren't afraid of a little hard work if it means you never have to diet again. Quick weightloss usually gives you saggy skin and then weight gain. Slow and steady weightloss with the right moderate exercises will help you tone up nicely and keep the weight off permanently. It will be more than worth it!

The other thing to keep in mind is that there has never been a harder time than now to try and lose weight properly. In fact, as time goes on, it will get harder and harder to get this right...again this is not your fault. What am I on about?

There has never been a time before in history where there have been this many choices for temptation than now. The junk available is sky high and will keep getting higher and higher. It is easier now more than ever before to fall off the wagon. More junk food can now be delivered to your door making it even more easy to grab your favourite take away and more companies are going digital with their advert campaigns. You can barely check your email without being spammed a picture advert for pizza. Using the Internet and clicking online leaves a footprint on the Internet, especially if you are using Facebook and social media. The videos you like and watch and the things you search for online slowly builds up and creates a database of who you are, what you like and what you dislike. That same pizza advert can now follow your footprints around the Internet, stalking you until you give in and order it! In 2012, fast food companies spent about US $4.6 billion on advertising. According to an article in The Guardian, research found that we are being bombarded with as many as 11 advertisements for junk foods during an hour's viewing of family-orientated television shows, such as X-Factor, The Simpsons and Hollyoaks. How can we contend with that? No wonder it is so hard to keep on the straight and narrow when our subconscious is being splashed with junk food everywhere we turn.

Think about our children, no wonder they are craving junk food. No wonder we have so many 'fussy eaters' who won't eat any veggies and instead opt for nuggets and chips all the time. None of this is our fault, but we need to be aware of what is out there and what our mind is being fed, if we want to overcome it and take back the control about what we feed our bodies. Not only that, but did you know these companies spend thousands on getting the taste JUST RIGHT to hit all the right spots in our brain to get us hooked? Junk foods are addictive. Remember the Pringles tag line, "Once you pop you simply can't stop"? Well, this isn't only a slogan. Junk foods like this are **scientifically** created to pinpoint parts of our brain connected to happy hormones to get us hooked. The mixture of fat, sugar, salt and MSGs in these junk foods are engineered for maximum taste, enjoyment and to keep us wanting more. With the combination of perfect advertising and scientifically tasty food, we really are up against it. If this wasn't enough to prove a point, try this little experiment out right now.

TO DO: Think of a nice hot fresh pizza. Think about how gorgeous the cheese is as you pull the slices apart. Imagine taking a bite and feeling your teeth sink into that melted cheese and pizza base. Close your eyes and visualise enjoying your pizza. Is your mouth watering yet? Maybe pizza isn't your thing. Visualise a doughnut, a croissant, pieces of chocolate…visualise your favourite junk food and notice how much you suddenly want it. How your mouth waters. How you need it right now and can't think of anything else.

Sorry to do that to you…writing that has made me want a pizza too, but I needed to prove a point! We are not always aware of the reactions our body has when we see or visualise these junk foods. We are well and truly hooked and sometimes it takes ALL of our efforts to resist thinking about junk food, let alone abstain from eating it. Again, none of this is your fault.

When you understand that 'the man' does not have your best interest at heart and in fact only YOU are in control of your weightloss and your health, the sooner you will start to see and feel the success you deserve. Be wise to what is going on around you. Understand, it is not you, it is them! Understand that you CAN take back the control.

This book consists of **3 Key Secrets** that you need to know if you want to lose weight and keep it off without dieting. I will be addressing some common myths most people believe to be true about dieting and weightloss and sharing the truth about them. Uncovering these myths will help you blast through the blocks standing between you and the body of your dreams.

The good news is we can help you finally lose weight and KEEP IT OFF... but before you get too stuck in to this book, take this quick test and find out if you are truly ready to quit dieting for good.

This matters to me a lot because you have to be ready. You have to really want this to work this time. It is the right thing for you only if you are ready for it because if you are, this can change your life. But if you are not, it will be a waste of your time and I will have offered you hope for nothing.

Take a moment to ask yourself the questions below. Score yourself one point for each YES.

- Are you really desperate to stop overeating?
- Do you hate the way your body looks most of the time?
- Does deciding what to eat feel like a minefield every day?
- Do you sometimes feel like a hopeless case?
- Do you feel you are out of control or have no willpower to make it work?
- Do you think about food (almost) all the time?
- Would you give just about anything to stop obsessing about food and your body?

- Would you say you are heavier now than when you went on your first diet?
- Have you tried Weight Watchers, Slimming World or other diet clubs more than once...or twice?
- Have you tried any of the other diets previously? (Cabbage soup, fasting, Atkins, Cambridge diet etc.)
- Are you prepared to do something that takes time and effort to get what you want?
- Are you open to receiving support, guidance and encouragement from kind people who actually understand and care about your success?
- Do you find yourself checking to make sure something is 'low calorie' or 'low fat?'
- Are you frustrated because you seem to have hit a plateau in your journey or are you consistently floating between a few different weights?
- Do you feel like you have tried it all and nothing works?
- Are you ready for something brand new unlike anything you have ever tried before?

How did you get on?

If you scored more than 5, it is time to make a change. Take a deep breath. It is time to forget everything you already know about weightloss. It is time to forget about the calorie counting and obsessing about numbers before you eat a meal. Take a weight off your shoulders and take the pressure off. It is time to stop feeling bad about yourself. It is time to stop feeling guilty about your cravings and what you eat.

Are you in?

Are you ready to try a new way?

Ready to know the truth about weightloss?

Are you ready for success?

Let's go!

CHAPTER 1: Secret #1

Eating more food is the key to losing more weight!

The idea that eating less food is the only way to lose weight, is the biggest myth the diet industry would have us believe to be true...this section is all about eating more food and not feeling guilty about it!

MYTH – You think you have to restrict calories, fats, carbs, syns, points, grams or other numbers to lose weight.

TRUTH – You need to start looking at the quality of the foods you eat rather than the quantity. The average amount of calories a woman needs each day is around 2000 (give or take a few here and there.) You can absolutely lose weight eating your 2000 calories a day instead of restricting yourself and eating less food and feeling hungry and grumpy in the process. The key is to start looking at WHAT you eat not how much, because not all calories are the same. For example, 2000 calories made up of pizza, crisps and cake will make you gain weight and gain fat. Whereas 2000 calories of real, whole foods like veggies, fruit, beans and pulses will give you overall better health and it will be easier for you to lose weight and fat. Another big thing is that low calorie, low syn or low points does not equal healthy or good for you. If you start looking at the ingredients of the food you eat and sticking to eating real foods – as much as possible – you will start to see shifts in your weight without restricting calories. Here is another example; low syn and low point processed foods are 9 out of 10 times higher in chemical additives, which can actually cause your body to store fat. When you start to embrace and understand that 200 calories of a homemade fruit and veg smoothie as a quick pick me up is better than 0 calories of a coke zero, you will start to see results. Calories are not the enemy. Calories are merely an energy substance. Energy our body needs to work effectively. The same way you will fill up the car with petrol to make it run, we need to fill our body with energy. Junk food contains what I call 'empty calories'...these are the calories that add to our daily calorie intake but are not very good sources of energy and have a low nutrient value. Empty calories are what we want to avoid but not all calories are bad. Let's not tarnish the good calories with the same brush as those naughty empty calories. It is the empty calories, which contribute to weight gain. The truth is we need calories, (energy), to survive and we can lose weight and keep it off without calorie restrictions and deprivation.

MYTH – You think you have to eat less and skip meals to maintain your weightloss results.

TRUTH – Skipping meals and eating less food for a long period of time actually slows your metabolism and makes your body store fat! Contrary to what you have been told, when we cut back on food, our body will slow its process of converting food into energy. Instead of the food, (calories), being used as an energy source, our body goes into something called starvation mode. This is where our body thinks you are starving it and instead of using the food as energy, it starts to store it as fat; much like a squirrel storing nuts in his cheeks. Our body doesn't want to use up the small amount of food you have given it as energy because it doesn't know when it will get more energy, i.e. your next meal. It stores the food as fat, like saving for a rainy day as protection against you starving it! Not only that, but when you skip meals you are far more likely to snack on junk in-between meals and over-eat on your next meal. You are more likely to have cravings and less likely to be strong enough to fight them! Talk about self-sabotage! Skipping meals is the perfect way to store fat and create havoc in your body.

So going forward, let's stop skipping meals and starving ourselves and instead plan 3 main meals a day, plus snacks in between if you feel hungry. Do not deny your body the food, energy and nutrients it needs for weightloss and good health. Can we pledge here and now never to skip a meal again? Okay, sometimes we have no choice with the busy lives we lead, but let's not forcibly starve ourselves in a bid to lose a few pounds.

MYTH – You think you have to miss out on all the foods you love to lose weight.

TRUTH – There is a healthy alternative to almost all foods you love! Fact! When we abstain from all things we love, we end up feeling resentful and miserable in the end. We feel like it isn't fair and everyone else is enjoying themselves and yet here we are, not allowed to eat any of the 'good stuff' and STILL not losing any weight! Eventually, we will cave in and have a little binge on all the stuff we promised ourselves we were giving up. A binge could be a day, a week or even months of blowing out. This is followed by feelings of guilt and self-hate for being weak and what good does that do? None. At. All! The only thing you will achieve by giving up all the foods you love is the feeling of loss and sadness. Instead, start to experiment on healthy alternatives to the foods you love. Let's have a go at a couple ideas.

Love chocolate? Try using raw cacao instead. Raw cacao has so many health benefits, including a great source of iron and calcium. In fact, 100g of cacao contains more calcium than cow's milk. Cacao is also scientifically proven to be a natural mood elevator, stimulating the release of serotonin, which makes us feel happier and more relaxed. In my home, we make chocolate energy balls and chocolate shakes, which certainly hits that chocolate spot when you need a fix.

Love crisps? How about making your own courgette crisps? Courgettes are an amazing source of vitamin K for healthy blood and bones, vitamin C to boost the immune system and potassium, which is good for the heart and brain. All the enjoyment of crunchy crispy goodness without the added saturated fat and chemical additives from actual crisps.

You can find some of our tasty treat recipes at the back of this book, don't panic! This is actually one of my favourite hobbies. We ask our clients to challenge us with their junk food cravings so we can come up with healthier alternatives. So, if you find your guilty pleasure is not included please contact me and we can get to work creating a healthier alternative for you, our contact details are at the back of this book too.

MYTH – You think you have to miss eating out with friends and family.

TRUTH – Similar to the missing out on foods you love, segregating yourself from social activities will leave you feeling resentful and more likely to give in and fall far away from the wagon. Yes okay, so eating out at Maccy Ds wouldn't be advisable, but there are plenty of restaurants where you can go and have a great time without feeling too guilty afterwards. Here are our top tips to lose weight without committing social suicide.

Top 3 tips on how to eat out – without the guilt!

1. Never eat the bread on the table. How many times at home do you eat 1 or 2 bread rolls before your meal? Now think about how many times have you done this while out at a restaurant? When the server asks if you want the bread, say no to that refined carb, empty calorie space

filler. You don't need it. It's that simple. A similar rule applies for the bottomless fizzy drinks. While it may save you money, it is unnecessary to have 2 or 3 glasses of fizzy pop over an hour or two. To be honest, I never drink my calories in soft drinks while out at a restaurant. Again that is usually your empty calories. I usually stick to still water, unless on the occasions where I am pretending to be fancy...that's when I go for the "Prosecco dah'ling".

2. Learn which restaurants offer healthier options. There are so many restaurants now that offer a healthier option. Zizzi's Italian for example, offers a really tasty dairy free cheese pizza, which has less saturated fat than a regular dairy cheese pizza. Nando's has the most amazing quinoa salad that is filling and full of amazing nutrients. They even have sweet potato chips instead of white potato chips, which are much healthier. Wagamama have lovely options to choose from too. Their tuna and quinoa (Seared Nuoc Cham Tuna on the menu) is yummy and the wide range of soups and broths are very tasty. My favourite place to go however, is Leon. They have gluten free, vegan and vegetarian options, as well as great choices for kids too. They use brown rice instead of white and the ingredients are sourced ethically. My go-to-meal at Leon is the sweet potato falafel box. Plan ahead when you go out. Review the menu online before you arrive and you will find that most restaurants have healthier options. The key to it is all in the planning. This way you can go out and enjoy a lovely meal with family and friends minus the guilt!

3. Make a decision to leave off the extras when they ask you to buy more! Not only will you save money but you will reduce those pesky empty calories. I used to work as a restaurant manager and we were trained on the importance of upselling to customers. It was my job to make sure all my staff were asking the guests if they wanted starters and sides, or if they wanted a double vodka coke instead of a single, or if they wanted a bottle of wine instead of a glass. Restaurants want to make as much

money as possible from one table sitting at a time, which is why they ask you if you want more of everything. Here is the truth. The meal you ordered is enough. You do not need the extras. Decide from the get go if you are having a starter OR a dessert, rather than both. Be strong and say no, when they ask you to order extras.

MYTH – You think all carbs are bad!

TRUTH – The truth is we need carbs to live! I actually find it hilarious when I hear people say they are cutting carbs to lose weight. (Sorry, not sorry!). Cutting all carbs out of your diet is a recipe for disaster. Carbohydrates are the body's primary source of energy. Cutting carbs entirely is like turning off the electricity but expecting your light to switch on and give you light. Much like calories, not all carbs are made the same. Carbs are demonized as the enemy, but did you know that fruit and vegetables are in fact called CARBS? Why would you cut out fruit and veg for weightloss? Let's clear that up so we can move forward with the right sort of carbs. The carbs we need to cut out for weightloss and weight maintenance are what's called refined carbs. These are the 'whites'; white bread, white rice and white pasta. Another example for refined carbs are those 'healthy' store cereals, cereal bars and muesli. They are usually full of sugar, which will sabotage your weightloss. Refined carbs are low in nutrients (which also makes them empty calories), low in fibre, they increase cravings, they don't keep us full for long and they spike your blood sugar level. These refined carbs are the carbs we want to cut. But we do NEED to eat some carbs on daily basis. The types of carbs we need are complex carbs such as fruits, veggies and pulses. Yes, they are all carbs, but they are good and we need them. Whole ancient grains such as spelt, kumut or rye and quinoa are complex carbs. Complex carbs are full of nutrients and fibre and they keep us full for longer, they naturally stimulate the metabolism and won't spike your blood sugar level as much. If you are wondering what a blood sugar level is. Let's break it down.

Blood sugar level refers to the amount of sugar in your blood. When we eat, certain foods have what is called a High GI level, which means it releases sugar into the blood very fast. This causes our blood sugar level to rise very fast and crash back down quickly afterwards. When our blood sugar rises very rapidly, our body releases happy hormones, which make us feel good and is also addictive. These foods that spike our blood sugar do not keep us full for long, the happy feeling soon wears off and we have what is called a sugar crash because our blood sugar then drops again. It is at this point we feel awful and we start to crave that happy feeling again in the form of more sugary refined processed food. We mindlessly eat more High GI food, which spikes our sugar level and starts the cycle again. Refined carbs and sugar filled sweets and drinks are all culprits of spiking our blood sugar level, but complex carbs do not spike our blood sugar in the same way. Yes, it raises our sugar level as it releases energy into our body, but these complex carbs will keep us fuller for longer and will not give us a crash or cause us to crave more junk foods. It is these complex carbs that give us the fuel and the energy that keeps us going.

Check out my gorgeous little diagram explaining the differences in types of carbs and their blood sugar responses. For me this is a real eye opener to how our body reacts to different foods.

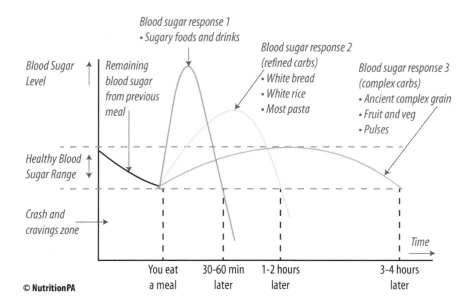

Blood sugar response 1
• Sugary foods and drinks

Blood sugar response 2
(refined carbs)
• White bread
• White rice
• Most pasta

Blood sugar response 3
(complex carbs)
• Ancient complex grain
• Fruit and veg
• Pulses

Blood Sugar Level

Remaining blood sugar from previous meal

Healthy Blood Sugar Range

Crash and cravings zone

Time

You eat a meal | 30-60 min later | 1-2 hours later | 3-4 hours later

© NutritionPA

Are we in agreement that carbs are a MUST? Without carbs our mind and body can't function properly. Some people will find short-term success by cutting carbs, but afterwards long-term weight gain! Other side effects from carb cutting can include headaches, feeling tired and weak, constipation or diarrhea. It is simply a case of choosing your carbs carefully. Now can you see why I find it amusing to see people say they are giving up all carbs? I am pretty sure you might find it amusing too the next time your BFF tells you they are cutting carbs. Spread the word and educate them about the differences in carbs and why it is crazy to think you can or should give them up entirely.

MYTH – You think you can – or you have to – do this alone.

TRUTH – This might be hard to hear for many people but I am a tough love person and I say this with my heart full of love for you. The truth is this; if you could have done this alone, you would have done it by now...and you wouldn't be reading this book. But you know what, that is absolutely okay. There is nothing wrong with getting help. For some reason, we think there are brownie points in saying, "I did this all by myself" which probably started in childhood. We were praised at school when we did it alone and scolded if we had a little look at someone else's correct answer. In adult life however, the tables turn. The people who get ahead and the people who have the most success are the people who get help and advice from someone a step ahead of where they are. Someone who is a professional in their field, someone who can guide them, and show them the way.

Here is a little secret. I am a qualified nutritional therapist and Health Coach and even I need some help to keep motivated with my own day-to-day diet sometimes. I am more than happy to admit that because it is okay to get help. I know I simply cannot be trusted around cake; it is that simple. Cake and me have had a long running turbulent relationship and all judgement goes out the window when cake shows up. It's like an abusive relationship. I KNOW it does me no good. I KNOW I feel awful afterwards but that doesn't stop me from going back for another slice. And another...and another...then another...and maybe a smaller slice next so I don't feel as bad...ahh, screw it I may as well finish the whole thing. I am more in control now than I used to be and have learned how to say no most of the time but it doesn't mean I am perfect and I have been known to go a little over board at times...especially in December! We are our own worst enemy and at times we need to accept help from people who can save us from sabotaging ourselves or beating ourselves up.

Here is another secret. Nearly every successful person today has had a coach or some sort of mentor, because the fact is most people need support and accountability to help them break through their blocks and self-doubt. Most of the time we don't even know we have blocks because we can't see them, where as someone else will see it and call it out. They will see it a mile off and help you move forward. You might not even want to hear it. You still might not see it at the time and the truth might hurt sometimes. But it **is** necessary to move forward. Not only that, but most people need accountability to make sure they follow through. Change is hard, but it's hardest when we are on our own because it is easier and more comfortable to slip into old habits. Having a coach to hold you accountable keeps you on your toes and to encourage you when times get rough. Yes, at times it will get rough, that is almost a given. You cannot expect your journey to always be a walk in the park and there will be times where you will feel like giving up and giving in but this is where a coach steps in.

"Accountability is the glue that ties commitment to the result."
Bob Proctor

Your Health Coach will hold you accountable and remind you of your goals, they boost you when you need it, they answer the technical nutrition and food questions about what to eat and they will guide you all the way to the finish line. They will hold your hand and be your cheerleader. Like having a personal trainer for all things fitness related, your Health Coach will help you in all things nutrition and health related. A coach can be the difference between success and failure. Having a coach is awesome and it makes this journey a whole lot easier and more fun too!

MYTH – You think having lists of 'good' and 'bad' foods is the answer to losing weight.

TRUTH – The truth is the food list is only the beginning. It scratches the surface but is only the very tip of the iceberg. It is a handy tool to have and a great place to start, but a list of what to eat and what not to eat simply isn't enough to get you across the finish line. The truth is deep down we all already know what to eat. We aren't stupid. We all know the basics of good and bad foods. We all know junk food when we see it, right? We all know sugar is bad but we eat it anyway! If I asked you what is the better option; cake or veggies, juice or fizzy pop? I am pretty sure you all know the answer. A list will not make your willpower any stronger than it is right now or stop you from eating the things you already know to be bad. Did you **know** that willpower accounts for a measly teeny tiny 7% of the decisions you make?

If you want to have long lasting success, you need to get an **education** about food and your body and how to deal with **emotional eating**. This goes much deeper than following a food list. Learning how food reacts in your body goes a long way to helping you make better decisions for yourself. My lovely blood sugar diagram from the previous page has achieved wonders for many clients who couldn't control their sugar cravings before. But seeing and understanding why you feel the way you do gives you more power to be able make better decisions. But even then it isn't easy because we have tendencies to choose food depending on our mood and how we feel emotionally at that time. Sometimes we have no idea we are eating emotionally until someone – a coach – points it out to us.

Seeing as we are on the subject of emotional eating, let's delve a little deeper. There are two main types of emotional eating.

1. We eat to celebrate or reward ourselves.
2. We eat because we feel sad, down, stressed or other negative emotions.

The first one is easier to start to overcome and let us begin with that. We are not dogs are we? Nope! So, let's make the conscious effort to stop rewarding ourselves with food. Again, this habit isn't our own fault. We usually learn how to reward ourselves with food from our family or parents or society at a very young age. Depending on how old you are you might remember being given a lollipop for being good at the dentist...I mean firstly, what a ridiculous reward for looking after your teeth, but secondly, this is a type of food reward we learn from a very young age. A friend of mine – who is usually very healthy – told me she took her daughter to a waffle and pancake place for having a good report at the end of Reception. For those who don't know, Reception age is 5 years old. Off they went and enjoyed a giant sized waffle and 4 large scoops of ice cream in one sitting. This might seem innocent, it is a treat after all and I am in no way calling anyone a bad parent for doing this. I have done it in the past and my parents have done it with me, but this is about opening our minds to break the bad habits, which get passed down from generation to generation. Not only is this type of food a recipe for disaster health wise, but this inadvertently teaches our kids one single lesson. Which is this; when **I am good I must reward myself with junk food and lots of it**! It might seem innocent because you want to make your child happy, but all we do is create a strong connection with junk food and happiness or junk food and rewards. In adulthood, this leads to nothing but disaster for most of us. Why teach our children how to get into this bad habit? The damage is already done for us as adults but we can choose to teach our children healthier habits from the start.

Food by nature is fuel. That is it. We eat to survive, to live and to stay alive. The purpose of food is not for enjoyment. I am not saying we cannot enjoy our food (anyone who knows me knows I certainly enjoy my food), but what happens over time is we begin to believe **food** = happiness, which is the downward spiral of emotional eating. Eventually we lose control and our subconscious takes over. As an adult, we start to eat without thinking, because in childhood the false belief was formed that food = happiness. It's not. It's fuel. Over time we can start to cut those emotional ties we have connected with food. We will enjoy having a cheat now and then but we won't be blindly turning to food as a reward or to make us happy.

There are many ways to stop rewarding ourselves with food. It takes time to break the habit but the food reward is easier to break because we are usually in a good mood when it happens, which means we have more control than when we are unhappy. We need to start by taking notice that we are doing it and then we can gradually change the routine.

Here is a little task we set for our clients who want to stop rewarding themselves with food.

TO DO: When you are in a good mood, write down 10 things you enjoy and make you happy that doesn't include any food or drink, things that you enjoy doing at home or out and about, alone or with friends. Do you like going to a spa? Do you enjoy painting? Do you love taking a bubble bath? Painting your nails? It is important to make sure you do this when you are in a good mood. When we are in bad moods or we have had a bad day, we are more likely to think negatively, which will make this task very difficult. When we are in a good mood this should be easy to think of 5 – 7 things, which make you happy and you enjoy doing. The next time you need to reward yourself for something, bring out your list instead of heading for the fridge or cupboards.

The second way we eat emotionally is when we feel sad or down. Do you remember my little blood sugar diagram? When our blood sugar spikes quickly (response number 1), our brain releases happy hormones into our body, which make us physically feel good and why it is only natural to reach for the junk foods to help us when we feel down. But do you know how to spot when you are emotionally eating?

Here is a little checklist for you to think about the next time you find yourself in the fridge or at the bakery section in the super market.

Real Hunger	Emotional Hunger
• Comes on gradually. • Can be satisfied with almost any food. • Once you are full you stop eating. • Causes satisfaction and no guilt.	• Comes on suddenly and feels urgent. • Causes specific food cravings such as ice cream, chocolate, crisps or pizza. • You eat more than you normally would and feel uncomfortably full. • Leaves you feeling guilty afterwards.

Start to notice what type of 'hunger' you are experiencing. We will be doing more work on emotional eating when we are uncovering Secret #3, but start to take note of the times you emotionally eat and see if you notice any patterns. When you are in that emotional zone, no amount of food lists can contend with that!

To sum up this section, I will leave you with a top tip, which brings together the concept of eating more food and having your cake and eating it.

Have a cheat meal!

Many of you have heard of the idea of cheat meals but what is it all about and how can you get in on it in a way that actually helps your weightloss results?

What is a cheat meal? A cheat is a meal where you let your hair down and eat whatever you feel like eating. Remember this is a cheat MEAL and not a cheat day. A lot of people (including me) make the mistake of having a whole day as a blowout, which is a recipe for disaster. Your cheat meal consists of a starter and a main or a main and dessert. I always opt for the latter – because I am slightly obsessed with desserts and all things sweet – as you may have picked up already.

How often can you indulge in your cheat meal? Your cheat meal is once a week if, and only if you feel like it and only have stuck to your plan all week. You need to have a plan of how you want your day-to-day diet to be and stick to it. Chances are if you haven't stuck to your plan then your cheat meal was inadvertently and accidently used up earlier in the week. All the more reason to stick to your plan, eh?

Why have a cheat meal? Cheat meals are great mentally and physically.

Mentally, they are fantastic because it means you can actually have your cake and eat it! It means you never have to give up chocolate again. You simply save it for your cheat meal instead. It means we don't have that feeling of depriving ourselves of everything we love and it reduces the cravings for those 'forbidden foods'. When they are no longer forbidden, you can eat what you want during your cheat meal without the feelings of guilt that creep up when you do something wrong. It is not wrong to enjoy a couple of slices of pizza and a glass of wine on an evening out with the girls. Once it is not wrong, you should no longer tolerate those feelings of guilt. I have a couple of friends who stress about the calories in their cheat meal. This is all kinds of crazy! The whole point of a cheat meal is to **ENJOY** it! What is the point of choosing the biggest main on the menu then talking about or worrying about the calories all the way through it? Eat it and enjoy it! It is also useful to us physically because it ramps up our metabolism and reduces the risk of plateau. A plateau is where you stop losing weight...for no apparent reason; it simply stops, which causes frustration. By having one planned cheat meal a week we can keep our metabolism on a roll and continue to lose weight gradually.

Any cheat pit falls to watch for? Learn from my mistakes. Don't have your cheat meal when you are starving hungry. This turns your organised cheat meal into a bingeing session and it will go from a nice celebration to you feeling overly stuffed and guilty afterwards. Your cheat meal should be a regular sized meal, not a mountain of junk because you are starving hungry. Plan your cheat meal in advance and eat on your plan for the rest of the day. Don't let emotions and starvations take over. This is especially important if you are planning on having your cheat meal at a dinner party. So many times we make the mistake of starving ourselves during the day because we know we are going out that evening. 'Saving ourselves' so to speak. This is a mistake because by the time it gets to the evening, all sanity goes out the window and you end up eating like there is no tomorrow, not because you lack willpower but because your body is hungry and crying out for you to feed it. Eat as you normally do in the daytime and by the time you hit the town on your big night out, you aren't starving hungry and are capable of making rational decisions regarding your cheat meal.

With that said...go and plan your CHEAT! Hurray!

CHAPTER 2: Secret #2

Working out more is not always the first step to boosting weightloss results

Abs are started in the kitchen BEFORE you hit the gym. This section is focused on all things fitness and exercise related.

MYTH – You think that you **must** work out **a lot** in order to lose weight.

TRUTH – The truth is unless you work out all day every day, you will **never** get the body you want **just** by working out! If you want to get that body of your dreams the most important change you will make is what you eat, your daily diet and lifestyle. Now don't get me wrong, I am not saying exercise isn't important because it is, but what you need to understand is that you will not lose weight and keep it off simply by working out 5 days in the gym, if you do not start with changing your diet. No, I do not mean go on a temporary diet. When I use the word diet, remember I am referring to what you eat day to day; your eating choices; and your lifestyle. Always remember when there is a big difference between going 'on a diet' and what you eat day-to-day, your diet for life.

Right, let's get back to the original myth about working out for weightloss. Let us have a look at this more closely. Some of you may be thinking, "But I have lost weight before at the gym though!" I am not saying you can't lose weight by vigorously working out in the gym, but similar to when you go on a faddy diet, when you go back to normal, so will your body. What you lost will creep back on at some point if you use extreme temporary methods. Unless you can keep up a high intensity level training for the rest of your life, it simply will not stick. You need to develop a workout routine that is something you can enjoy 2 – 4 days a week. Something you can stick to and keep yourself fit and give you a healthy heart into old age. The trouble is, many women are using working out as a way for them to continue to eat what they want or as a punishment for falling off the dieting wagon.

"Yes, I will have another slice of pizza today and then I will work out longer in the gym next week". Sound familiar? When exercise is used in this way, we will always be fighting a losing battle, rather than creating the body of our dreams. You are much more likely to stay exactly the same if you do not change your diet along with it. In some cases we have known people to actually gain more fat when they start working out, why? Because we as a society have been lead to falsely believe that working out is a free pass to eat whatever you want. It is not.

A 2006 study published in the *International Journal of Obesity* looked at 13,000 male and female runners and found that regular runners who were not overweight got heavier during a 17 year period if the amount of exercise they did remained the same. Shockingly, only those who **increased** their exercise intensity were able to prevent from gaining more fat.

What does this mean? It means that the key to sustainable weightloss is more than hitting the gym. Working out should be the icing on the cake, not the cake itself. It is the finishing touches and not the first move.

Your journey to better health and permanent weightloss will begin with changing your diet. Exercise is a bonus add-on to boost your results and not what you do because you feel 'fat' or to 'work off' what you ate.

MYTH – You think a personal trainer can tell you what foods to eat to lose weight and get healthy.

TRUTH – Want to hear the real truth about this; cold hard facts? This is gonna be hard for some people to grasp and is something very few personal trainers will openly admit. Here is the truth.

By law, a Personal Trainer is not permitted to give you in-depth advice on what foods to eat. Unless they have done the relevant add-on qualifications, they simply aren't licensed or insured to be giving in depth recommendations. To be clear I am in no way discrediting what Personal Trainers do, they are amazing! However, I have myself enrolled onto the Basic Level 3 Personal Training course and seen it for myself. The nutritional information within the Personal Training course is no way enough to be able to give substantial nutritional advice in any way shape or form. It also doesn't cover the best advice for health conditions such as Crohns or Thryroidism, for example. Personal Trainers work on numbers. For example, they can share with you how many grams of fat, carbs and proteins to eat and tell you how many calories to consume to get X result. However, they are not trained in exactly what foods do to your body while they are digesting or the dangers of GMO foods or pre-packaged processed meats and foods. While they can help your weightloss journey and give you a rough guide, they won't be able to delve into what is really healthy for you long term, unless they have completed an add-on nutrition qualification.

A previous flatmate of mine was a Personal Trainer and a very good one at that. One day she decided to compete in a fitness competition and she hired a trainer to help her who specialized in competitions. However, the outcome was far from desirable. This trainer had successfully competed himself and helped other people many times, but my friend was a vegetarian with specific needs and requirements. The trainer basically advised her to hardly eat any food, no fruit, no fats, not anything it seemed and as a result she was tired and grumpy all the time and in the end she couldn't continue his program and didn't even get to compete in the competition at all. The advice she was given was dangerous to her health and what made it worse was that she didn't end up reaching her end goal either, so it was all for nothing. While this trainer was the best in his field for fitness, he simply didn't have enough knowledge of food and nutrition to offer healthy or safe advice about what to eat.

Here's an example of acceptable and unacceptable nutritional comments in a hypothetical situation between a Personal Trainer and a client (from a presentation at the American College of Sports Medicine, Orlando, Florida, USA, April, 2006).

Acceptable: "Orange juice is a good source of vitamin C."

Not Acceptable: "You should drink more orange juice."

A small but clear difference. The acceptable comment is statement of fact. The second is recommendation.

What **CAN** Personal Trainers help you with then?

Having a Personal Trainer is great and they can offer amazing insights to help you achieve your fitness goals.

They can show you how to exercise CORRECTLY and SAFELY. Believe it or not, there is actually a right way and a wrong way to exercise. A Personal Trainer can do the necessary checks and give the correct advice for YOU. It is always good to remember that what might be good for you, may not be good for your friend with a bad back or weak knees, or after giving birth. Whatever advice a Personal Trainer gives you should be yours and yours only. They will assess YOUR abilities and any weaknesses to create a work out plan specifically for you. Refrain from getting together with buddies and sharing the tips your trainer gave **you** for **your** ears only.

They can show you how to build muscle and tone up. Personal Trainers are masters at manipulating our muscles. They will show you exactly what you need to do to tone the places you want to tone and get rid of those pesky wobbly bits. They can literally sculpt your perfect body with their genius moves, (along with your change of diet of course).

They can show you how to use the gym equipment. The equipment in the gym can be very dangerous when not used correctly. If you are having a session in a gym, the Personal Trainers are on hand to make sure you are using everything correctly. They can also show you what gym equipment will work which muscles. I always notice women jumping on the treadmill and cross trainer when they hit the gym. In reality, the results you are looking for probably won't come from those machines.

They can give you a rough guide on how many fats, carbs, proteins and calories to eat depending on your height and weight. According to official guidelines, there is a certain recommendation of how much of each component you need depending on your personal body statistics. While this can be a good place to start your journey as we discovered earlier, not all calories or carbs are equal and the same goes for fats and proteins. There are certain foods that offer good fats we need and certain foods that offer fats that are damaging to our health. Being advised to simply have X amount of fats is not sufficient enough to guarantee weightloss or good long-term health. I have a very good Personal Trainer friend of mine who openly admitted she had one client who needed extra fat according to her statistic counting. The first thing she knew would fill that exact amount of fat requirement was to recommend a bag of crisps! Luckily enough she had the common sense to ask me what she could offer instead, but there are some Personal

Trainers who simply do not know enough about food to be able to offer the best advice and the healthiest alternatives. The best thing you can do is to stick with them for the fitness advice, but ask someone qualified in nutrition for food advice. As a nutritional therapist and ex-professional dancer, I like to think I know about keeping fit and being healthy. But it is not my expertise nor am I qualified in fitness, so you won't catch me trying to offer in-depth fitness advice to my clients, even though I know a lot about keeping fit. It would be irresponsible for me to offer fitness advice, as it would be for a Personal Trainer to offer in-depth nutrition advice.

They can show you WHICH exercise and workouts are best for you depending on your personal fitness goals. Here is another reason the advice they give you should be yours and yours alone. Your Personal Trainer not only knows the safest way for YOU to exercise based on your strengths and weaknesses, but they also know the most effective way for you to reach YOUR specific fitness goals. If your friend's goal is to get a nice bum and her Personal Trainer gives her bum exercises, there is no point you copying her to reach your goal of getting abs of steel. Different exercises will help you reach different goals, which is why it is important for you to have your own session rather than do whatever your mate is doing.

MYTH – You think having a gym membership is going to make you exercise and reach your goal.

TRUTH – That's the story we tell ourselves to make us feel better for not doing what we know we should have been doing. We realise we haven't been doing our best and we run out (in good faith) and join a class or gym. It feels like a sense of accomplishment or we have done something for the greater good. But in truth, no amount of memberships will **make** us actually show up. The truth is, it is easier **not** to exercise. I speak for myself and many other women I have spoken to in the same dilemma where they really want to get fit, but deep down can't be bothered! Can't be bothered to leave the sofa on a rainy Saturday afternoon or get up 2 hours early to get a routine in before heading into work. It is hard there is no denying. Then, when we actually get to the gym, we wonder around without a clue of what we are doing. I usually spend far too long fixing my hair in the changing rooms. My ponytail has to be perfect for the treadmill you know! Not too high and not to low, will make it swing from side to side as I jog...Yes that is actually the type of thing I think about at the gym rather than getting down to it!

However, the key to make us more willing to get to the gym and actually exercise is having a plan! Knowing what we want to achieve and knowing exactly how to do it. Knowing how to use the equipment. Knowing how many of each squat and sit-up we should be doing. Knowing the different types of squats and sit-ups to do and when to do them. Knowing how to keep our routines fresh and exciting so we don't get bored and want to hang ourselves mid-session. It is the confidence of having a plan and knowing what we are doing that makes all the difference. This is where a Personal Trainer comes in perfectly. They will do all the hard work so we don't have to. They will figure out what exercises, how many and when to do them. They give us the plan to help us achieve our goal!

The other thing to bear in mind is that not everyone was meant to get fit in the gym! Don't waste your money signing up because you think that you **should**, but deep down know it isn't actually what you want. No one said the only way to be physically fit was to join a gym. We have been fed this false ideal of what working out is **meant** to look like, but the truth is not everyone's vision needs to be the same. Yours doesn't need to be the same as your friends or your neighbor. This is your journey not theirs. We spend too much of our lives trying to do what we think we **should** be doing and in the meantime we miss out on other amazing experiences. Not anymore. You have permission to be free! Stop trying to fit in and do things that other people are doing because you feel obligated to. You know when I said I spent more time in the changing room than actually working out, that's still true to this day. I feel sick thinking about the gym. I am bored to death right now even talking about the gym. I've rolled my eyes about 10 times writing this and right now I am actually shaking my head at how BORING THE GYM IS! The gym isn't my thing and that is absolutely okay. I am a dancer and my preferred form of exercise is dance. I like ballet. I like pop. I like tap. I love dance. Give me a studio, a barre for stretching and some music and I am off! What do you love? Pilates? Yoga? Pole dancing? Take your pick. But whatever you choose make it something you absolutely love and enjoy. This is the best way to ensure you are actually going to get up off your arse and do it!

MYTH – You think weightlifting is for guys and will make you look like a man.

TRUTH – Lifting weights is the best! Remember when I was talking about the fact that most women end up on the cross fit thing and treadmill? While they have their place, the truth is lifting weights makes you strong, toned and sexy and no, you will not look like a man...unless of course that's your goal. But it would take an awful lot of effort for the average woman lifting average weights to end up looking like a guy. The bottom line is no matter how far you run and no matter how little you eat those bingo wings aren't going anywhere until you pick up some weights. Remember this should be organised by a Personal Trainer! Take it from me; my arms are stick thin. They always have been and never have much fat as my fat goes to my legs, bum and tum. But even little skinny arms like mine will have bingo wings if I don't pick up some weights and keep them toned. We have flesh all over our body. We can choose that flesh to be saggy fat or we can choose that flesh to be toned muscle. Simply doing cardio and eating less food won't create toned muscle, it will reduce the fat yes but we need to lift weights in order to gain the muscle.

Here are 4 really cool benefits of lifting weights.

1. Weight training can help to improve your posture and reduce back pain because it strengthens your core, which will help you stand taller with a straighter spine.

2. While weight training builds muscles, it also strengthens your bones too and can reduce the risks of osteoporosis, fractures and broken bones.

3. Many women have this fear they will look big, bulky and man-like, but actually most of us ladies don't have it in us to get that bulky because we simply don't have the testosterone men do. Women have about 20 times less testosterone then men. This means that when we lift, instead of getting big and bulky, us women develop strength and gorgeous definition without the size.

4. Weight training will boost your metabolism! Yes really. As we gain more lean muscle, our body goes into overdrive burning more fat. The more lean muscle we have the more our body wants to burn fat. Studies have found that the average woman who weight trains 2 to 3 times a week for 2 months will gain nearly 2 pounds of muscle and will lose 3.5 pounds of fat and over time this will really add up! More muscle equals less fat! Hurrah!

You see, lifting weights is not only good for guys, it is good for all of us. If, like me, you don't fancy the gym, you can grab some dumbbells online or pop into Argos! Start off light and then get advice from a Personal Trainer to take it further.

Let's sum up this section about exercise and fitness. What are my biggest take always from this subject?

Don't wing it. Your exercise routine needs planning!

Set Your Goal

Like most journeys in life, you need to know your end goal. Simply saying you want to lose weight is very vague. Lose weight where, your forehead or your thighs? Know what you want, don't just wing it. How many dress sizes or inches are you wanting to go down? Are you wanting to get a firm bottom or maybe what's behind you doesn't matter to you and you want abs of steel instead? Whatever you decide, make sure you know your goal and write it down. Goals written down are more likely to be achieved.

Do your homework before signing up to a gym

Once you have set your goals and made a plan of what you want to achieve, do your homework before jumping into a gym membership. You need to make sure the gym provides what you want and what you will enjoy. If you love swimming, does it have a pool? If you love yoga, do they offer yoga classes within your membership? If not, how much extra per class is it? If it works out a lot more expensive, perhaps joining a yoga studio would be more beneficial? Shop around. Ask for a gym tour. Do they have a sauna for you to relax in? Make sure you know what you want out of your gym relationship. If it doesn't offer what you want, don't be pressured into signing up and explore other options.

Find a personal trainer who you connect with and who specializes in what YOU want to achieve and ask for a FREE TRIAL SESSION or CLASS.

Working in the health industry, I meet a lot of people who work in the fitness industry. All the best class teachers, fitness instructors and personal trainers I personally know give a trial session free of charge before requesting a payment. You need to make sure your teacher or trainer knows their stuff and can motivate you too. You need to have a connection with them, which will really help you want to keep going to the gym or class. If your trainer rubs you up the wrong way, you are more likely to want to skip sessions or skip classes to avoid them. Now, I am not saying you need to be best buds, but you need to like them enough to stay with them for the long term. They also need to have the necessary qualifications to help you for anything specific. For example, if you have had a baby, not any trainer will do. You need a trainer who has been qualified in post-natal exercise. Ask questions and see how they fit in with your requirements and your goals. Just like with the gym, don't be afraid to shop around.

Work with your trainer and ask questions about how you can continue at home

Once you have chosen a trainer for you, be it in a gym, class or an outside trainer, ask them how you can continue at home. Unless you have insane goals like bodybuilding or marathon training, you shouldn't really need to see your trainer more than 2 or 3 times a week. Having a trainer shouldn't need to cost you an arm and a leg because they request you to be with them 5 days a week. A good trainer will be more than happy to give you routines or exercises to do in between sessions either in the gym or at home.

CHAPTER 3: Secret #3

Diet foods, weightloss groups and diet companies are like wolves dressed in sheep's clothing and are setting us up for failure rather than success.

We are finally on Secret #3 and as you can see from the title, it's a biggie! I touched on this in the introduction and this section will really start to bring everything together. Are you ready?

MYTH – You think there is a specific timeline in which you should get your results.

TRUTH – The hard truth is, until you have done it and reached your goal, there is no way of telling how quickly or slowly you will reach your desired results. All of those adverts for X amount of day challenges you see which guarantee you will lose so many pounds or kilos in so many days or weeks are quite simply having us all on! You will find most of them will have something in their small print saying they can't guarantee any results...but who reads the small print right? You get all excited, jump in and expect those results...then when they don't come, we end up feeling like failures. Yes, of course, some people will reach the goal in the said number of days but not everyone. We are not all made up exactly the same way and what works for your BFF or your neighbour might not work for you in the same time frame. Plus, we also have to remember that we do not know what goes on behind closed doors. A friend who is seeing results quickly, might not have the same temptations as you. They might not be dealing with emotional eating the way you are. They might be younger than you. They might have a healthier gut than you and people with healthier guts can often lose weight faster than those with unhealthy guts. There are so many variables. We are all different. We must never compare. Your journey is your journey. These false advertising campaigns are set up to make us feel like we are failing because when we don't reach that goal like someone else did, what happens? We feel like a failure and most of the time we are too embarrassed by our apparent 'failure' that we never say anything about it. We never go back to them and say, "Hey you! I didn't lose what you said I would in 3 weeks!" Oh no. Instead we stand in front of the mirror and say to ourselves, "Hey you! You're a failure!" Then we continue to walk around thinking we are no good.

Hear this right now from me. Know, like you know, like you know, that it is **not** your fault. Those kinds of challenges are set up to make us feel like it's our fault so we come back out of desperation to try them again, then again and again. But now we know, don't we? It is not us, it's them.

MYTH – Your think results are measured by checking your weight on a set of scales

TRUTH – Cue a big red flashing light and loud horn sign – Newsflash – The scales LIE to you! They are your worst enemy. They are evil and you mustn't believe what they say to you! Yet, what happens at almost all diet clubs? We check in each week to get weighed! It makes me want to scream.

The number on the scale will never take the time or care to consider your time of the month, how much muscle you have, that pint of water we drank or if you have done a poo that day! When we have our period we are usually heavier than normal. After we have done a poo we can sometimes be lighter. After we drink a pint of water we will be heavier. Did you know if you weigh yourself on a Monday morning, you are statistically more likely to be heavier than on a Friday morning? Any guesses why? The weekend is when we usually have a cheat meal, attend birthday parties and generally let ourselves go a little, so statistically we will usually be heaviest after the weekend. All you ladies who get up on a Monday morning and begin their week with a weight check, the scales have fooled you into thinking you have made less progress than you probably have overall. There are many variables when it comes to how much we weigh at any given time and the scales are not an accurate tool to measure success. There are too many ups and downs within a day or a week, which the scale isn't capable of accounting for.

The scales make me genuinely angry when I think about all the times we as women are made to feel like we are failing on 'weigh-in day' at the weightloss group or slimming club because the numbers aren't what we wanted them to be. Lose a pound, gained a pound; lose a kilo, gained a kilo. You sit around watching the other women get their little certificates of weightloss and here you are feeling like a big fat failure. What we don't realise is some of those women don't eat all day to make sure their weigh in goes to plan. Yet, in that moment when they are rejoicing, we are left hating ourselves even more. I used to feel like I was going nowhere and all my hard work was for nothing. But do you know what I figured out one day? The more the numbers were rising, the more working out I did, the more working out I did, the more muscle I was gaining and guess what...the higher those scales were! Fact! Muscle weighs more than fat in terms of density and size. I see the confusion so many times when people say, "But a tonne of anything is still a tonne, right?" Not in terms of size. If you had 1 kilo of peanuts and 1 kilo of oranges, they would both weigh 1 kilo but you would have many more peanuts than you would have oranges because oranges are bigger than peanuts. The oranges take up more space. A kilo of muscle takes up far less space than a kilo of fat in your body. Therefore, technically it absolutely will weigh more than fat in your body. PLUS muscle is an **active** tissue. Remember what we learned in the weight lifting section. More muscle means better and faster metabolism, which also means more fat loss.

Check this out... another of my wonderful diagrams for you to enjoy.

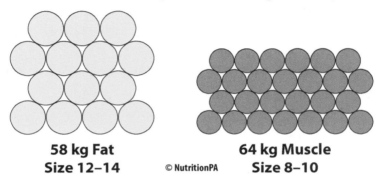

58 kg Fat   © NutritionPA   **64 kg Muscle**
Size 12–14   **Size 8–10**

The squares represent your stunning before and after photos. It took me ages to get it right, I hope you can see the resemblance. In your before photo you weigh 58kg on the scales. In your **after** photo you think you look pretty good but when you step on the scale you weigh 64kg which is MORE than you did before. If you were to trust those scales as a measurement of your success, how would you be feeling after working out and eating right? Here you are on weigh-in day and you do not weigh less but you weigh more than you did to start with! Would you be celebrating with your biggest loser certificate or would you start to feel like you are failing and wonder what's gone wrong? My guess is most people would be feeling pretty deflated. Deflation usually leads to a fall or a jump off the wagon, which undoes all of your hard work. I have actually known people who have quit their work out program because the scales weren't reflecting their success and as a result ended up regaining all the fat they had previously lost. How sad is that? Imagine thinking you are failing when actually in reality you are winning! Makes me want to cry thinking about it.

However, if you use other ways to measure your success instead of or as well as the scales you will immediately start to see your progress and feel amazing, instead of crappy. Dress size is a great way to measure progress. In your **before** photo you are a size 12 – 14 and in the **after** photo an 8 – 10. This shows your success plainly and simply. By the way, I am not saying your goal should be an 8 – 10 dress size, this is an example only because it was my first initial goal. Another way you can measure yourself is with a tape measure, how many inches have you lost? My favourite way to measure my progress is with a body fat % machine. Now that I have reached my goal of a size 8 on top and a 10 on the bottom, most of the time my dress size stays pretty much the same, but the most accurate way for me to check further progress is with a body fat % machine. Your gym may have one of these but if not, most of the larger Boots stores have them. Whatever you decide to do to measure your success is up to you, but please stop relying on scales and scales alone. Are we all in agreement that the scales are not our friends, anymore? Fab, let's burn them and move on.

MYTH – You think light, low fat, low calorie and diet foods are good or healthy.

TRUTH – The truth is the majority of light, low fat or diet foods are terrible for our overall health and what is worse is that many of them will sabotage your weightloss results! Here's the scoop.

When the low fat guidelines first came about, many of the food manufacturers jumped on the bandwagon and wanted a piece of the – low fat – pie; the money! They wanted to bring 'healthy' low fat foods to the market, to sell to the ever-growing health conscious consumer. However, what they discovered was a big FAT problem. Yes, a little pun to make me laugh, these are for my own enjoyment, but I hope you find them amusing too? The issue they found is that when you remove fat from foods meant to have fat in them, they end up tasting HORRIBLE! To deal with this, the food manufactures had to get clever (sneaky). To make foods taste yummy again they added sugar, sweeteners and other toxic chemicals instead. Sugar is not a fat it is a carbohydrate. Therefore, a product can be labelled 'low fat' even though it is loaded with sugar. 'Low fat' foods lowers our guard and tricks us into thinking we are eating something good for us, which, in turn usually means we end up eating more of it than we mean to. The added refined sugars will lead to blood sugar spikes, followed by crashes and cravings, making it more difficult to control our overall food intake and food choices. This means the third or fourth 'low fat' biscuit starts to look very tempting! We think, "Ooh it's low fat? I'll have another one then!" But a diet too high in these 'low fat' products can be as unhealthy as a high-fat diet because it increases the risk of diabetes, heart disease and causes high cholesterol levels as well as more weight gain! YIKES! While initially people can lose weight eating diet foods, they will almost always put the weight back on or hit a brick wall in their journey.

The best example and my personal pet hate are a certain brand of light yogurts. I won't name them for now. But let us call them Yogurt X. Many of these are low syn and low calorie and for this reason I have known people on 'diets' eat 2 or 3 of them in a row. For those of you wondering, a syn is a measurement from a popular diet club; they count syns rather than calories. While these Yogurt X's may taste yummy, they are not a health food as we are lead to believe. Did you know one pot of strawberry Yogurt X, contains 10.6 grams of sugar which converts to more than 2 ¼ teaspoons of sugar? But I thought they said it was light? Well, it's not light in sugar that's for sure! Think about it. We could easily have 2 pots of these a day because they have no fat, only 99 calories and no syns at all leading us to believe they are healthy...but actually 2 of these have the equivalent amount of sugar as 6 chocolate digestive biscuits (that's nearly half the pack by the way!) Just in 2 small pots of 'low fat', 'diet', 'healthy', 'calorie free', strawberry Yogurt X. No wonder we find it so hard to shift the weight if we are eating all this low fat rubbish.

Now I know what you might be thinking. But it has no fat, we won't get fat if we don't eat fat...guess again. Thinking fat makes you fat is like thinking strawberries will make you red and oranges make you orange. Remember the blood sugar diagram, remember that refined sugar makes our blood sugar spike, which will be followed by a crash and a craving for more refined sugar. Sugar is usually the main reason why we struggle to lose weight. We know how to avoid saturated fat, that's the easy part. We know fried food is the bad kind of fatty. We know doughnuts and cakes are fatty. But sugar sneaks in usually where we least expect it and we over consume sugar in things that we believe are healthy such as all those low fat, light foods. The ingredients lists are usually confusing too. I am a health professional with training in how to read a food label, but it took even me a while to figure it out and I had to use a calculator too! But get this, on the Yogurt X label it stated only 7.1 g of sugar for a serving of 100 grams, but the pot itself was 175 grams, which can be easily misunderstood or overlooked. Actually in every pot we end up consuming more sugar than we think we are. Per pot it is not 7.1 grams of sugar as the label would lead us to believe, it is actually more than 10 grams of sugar because it is 175g, which is nearly double the started figure that we see on the pot. That is also nearly half of the Daily Recommended Allowance of sugar according to the National Health Service, taken up by simply **one** tiny yogurt! Unless you have a good grip of quick mental maths, who will actually have the time and patience to stand in the cold fridge aisle of the supermarket and work this stuff out? Not many people! Oh, and on a side note, sugar is not only going to spike your blood sugar levels, it has also been proven to accelerate the growth of cancer cells. Then, to add insult to the already injured, these diet foods also contain artificial ingredients too! This Yogurt X contains aspartame as well as sugar. Aspartame is one of THE worse artificial sweeteners on the market and is a known carcinogen and neuro toxin, which means it is linked to cancer and is toxic to our brains. Oh and like most other artificial sweeteners it has also been linked to weight gain since the 1980s! This is not new information because these are facts going back to when I was still in nappies! Yes, I am an 80s baby and proud! The trouble is that we aren't educated about these facts. We have to take control for our own health and learn about these things.

So, here we are on our 'diet', trying to be healthy eating all this low fat, low calorie, low syn, light diet foods, (recommended by a diet group leader with no health or nutritional qualifications), which are actually more likely to help us put on weight rather than lose it and could potentially damage our health long term. Here is my advice, if you are going to eat 2 light diet yogurts to lose weight, you may as well have half a pack of chocolate biscuits. Both are unhealthy. Neither will help you lose weight but as at least with the biscuits you **know** what you're getting. You already **know** they are unhealthy, which means you are less likely to keep eating more and more of them while thinking they are good for you and PLUS; and here is the kicker, they usually contain less sugar and less toxic chemical too!

The bottom line is AVOID light, low fat, diet and low calorie foods like your life depends on it because in reality, your life does depend on it! Diet foods are usually hidden with loads of toxic nasties, artificial rubbish, as well as higher amounts of SUGAR, which are fundamentally damaging to your long-term health.

This also includes most of the packaged stuff you find in the 'healthy' section in the supermarket. Cereal bars, diet cereals, packaged diet meals etc. are included in this section. Check the labels and most of the time they are very low in nutrients and high in sugar and artificial ingredients, which means they are empty calories! They won't keep you full for long and will encourage more junk food cravings...oh and leaves you feeling hungry again very quickly.

MYTH – You think meal replacement shakes, protein powders and smoothies are a great way to lose weight.

TRUTH – Unfortunately, most store bought smoothies and shakes contain high amounts of sugar and artificial ingredients just like the low fat diet foods in the last myth. Let's get dug in and have a look at the ingredients of a very popular high street meal replacement shake.

> *Sugar, High Oleic Sunflower Oil, Maltodextrin, Gum Arabic, Milk Protein Concentrate, Cellulose Gel, Soy Fibre, Buttermilk Powder, Potassium Phosphate, Xanthan Gum, Dextrose, Salt, Guar Gum, Soybean Lecithin, Artificial Flavor, Carrageenan, Sodium Phosphate, Acesulfame Potassium (A Non Nutritive Sweetener) and Aspartame.*

It doesn't take a rocket scientist to see there is nothing nutritious on this list, yet we are being sold this as a suitable replacement for a nutritious meal by a very well-known company, which you have probably used and may be still using right now. This is simply wrong and in my opinion should be banned! The ingredients above are NOT a suitable replacement for a well-balanced and nutritious meal. The first ingredient is sugar and remember we know about sugary drinks and blood sugar levels. The next ingredients are all highly processed or chemicals and artificial sweeteners. There is absolutely nothing good in this shake whatsoever. It genuinely makes me angry when I see women piling their baskets with this stuff under the impression they are making a good and healthy choice. I have visions of running into the supermarket with a balaclava on and smashing all the shelves with this crap on it and then jumping up and down – like a mad woman – on these products so people stop buying them! The trickery and clever marketing is just so insane. Again, this is not your fault. It is not you, it's them. Stay away. Avoid them like the plague.

Protein powders

Some protein powders are amazing but others are a straight up mess dressed in pretty packaging. It is so important to always, always read the label but to read the label effectively you need to know what you are looking for. I see so many people in the supermarket picking up products and glancing at the back like they know what it all means. I'm not judging, I used to do it myself. I would stand there with the item in my hand reading all the big words at the back and nodding my head intelligently because I wanted to take control over what I was feeding myself and my family. But deep down I knew I only understood half of what was written and what is worse, even if I understood the word, I didn't really know if it was a good or bad ingredient. This is where education is the key. The more educated you are the easier it will be to know what you are looking for in food and protein powders too! Choosing the right protein powder is tricky but here are a few tips to get started.

Most people these days are using protein powder, not only after working out, but in their smoothies too. While the added protein does have many benefits, the TYPE of protein you use is very important.

The most popular choice is Whey Protein, yet most people have no idea where whey really comes from. So, here it is. Whey is a bi-product of the cheese manufacturing process. It used to be known as curds and whey and was classed as nothing more than WASTE, until one day, some smart alec discovered its high protein content.

While it is indeed high in protein, it can also have a negative impact on our health. Firstly, it's a dairy product. We actually lose the enzyme we need to break dairy down effectively while we are still children. As a result, most of the population are lactose intolerant and don't realise it. Think about it. How many people do you know in adult life who have suddenly become lactose intolerant? Don't you think the amount of lactose intolerant people in general is much more than it was 10 years ago, say? This is because instead of suffering with the symptoms, more and more people are getting tested and diagnosed. Whether you are intolerant or not, eating high amounts of diary can put added pressure on our digestive systems. Secondly, whey absorbs very quickly and has been proven to spike your blood sugar level. This might be good for some people post-workout, but using this in a meal replacement shake is a disaster move. Consuming whey (diary), can lead to acne breakouts, weight gain, as well as gut problems including bloating and Irritable Bowel Syndrome.

Soy protein is also very popular, but not the best option because it can mimic the female hormone; estrogen. Our hormones play a key part in weightloss and consuming soy can in fact contribute to weight gain! Other side effects include early menopause in ladies and low sperm count in men. The other reason to avoid soy is because it contains chemical compounds called goitrogens, which can affect negatively the thyroid. Our thyroid controls how fast or slow your body uses energy, in other words it controls your metabolism. Slow metabolism means slower weightloss.

The best protein to use is a plant-based protein such as pea or hemp protein for example. Unlike whey, pea and hemp protein is naturally cholesterol free and fat free and can actually aid in weightloss, BINGO!

What else to look out for?

The other thing to look out for in your protein powder is the added sugars and sweeteners, including sucrose and fructose, as well as other artificial ingredients. Most products contain some sort of sugar to make it taste better, but the **type** of sugar makes all the difference. Natural sugars like stevia or cane sugar are going to be better options than any of the artificial sugars. You want to choose a powder that is as PURE as possible, which is why we only use and recommend one brand. The brand we use are free of artificial flavours, colours and sweeteners, gluten free, vegan certified and is jam packed with 20 essential vitamins and minerals including Coenzyme Q10, which is perfect for anti-aging from the inside out! Hurray! If you want to know more about proteins and meal replacements, feel free to get in touch and we can share more about this. It really can be a whole new world of excitement!

Smoothies

Store bought smoothies are pretty much a no-no all round. Not to say we should never have them and of course there are exceptions, but on the most part they are not a healthy choice of beverage. The most popular smoothie brand is actually the worst offender. Let's have a look. There is nothing 'innocent' or 'healthy' about these smoothies. This is clever marketing at its best! These teeny tiny little smoothie bottles can contain up to 34.4 grams of sugar which is equivalent to 3 and a half Krispy Kreme doughnuts or in other words EIGHT AND A HALF teaspoons of sugar. WOWZERS! That is 30% more sugar than a coca cola. 250ml of not so much fruit smoothies is your entire recommended daily sugar allowance and then some more on top. Need we go any further? Let's simply say, you are far better off grabbing an apple instead of a store bought smoothie.

But what about the humble homemade smoothie? These are great IF you make them correctly. I call home made smoothies my 'number one miracle method' because they give results. I've had clients do nothing else other than substitute a protein packed smoothie for their breakfast and they lost weight faster and burned more fat!

High-protein foods curb your appetite and keep you full longer. A protein-rich breakfast suppresses hunger far better than a carbohydrate heavy breakfast. That's why a protein and fruit and veg smoothie can be the perfect solution for breakfast or an afternoon snack.

However, not all smoothies are made equal. To really benefit from your smoothie, you'll want to design it correctly. I don't want you making the mistakes I made, which crash-and-burn an otherwise healthy attempt to lose weight. Not only that, but a smoothie with the wrong ingredients can actually make you put on weight rather than lose it! YIKES! Imagine that, all your hard work ruined for the sake of some badly built smoothies. Let's make sure we get this right!

Top mistakes when making homemade smoothies, with solutions for you.

1. Turning your smoothie into a sugary fake shake.

Mistake: One of the biggest smoothie making mistakes is when we blend fruit with fruit and more fruit. Then to top it off, we go and add high sugar ingredients like sugary dried fruit, sweetened milks, nut butters with added sugar, chocolate powder etc. This can easily turn a potentially healthy smoothie into a sugar-loaded, fat-storing disaster.

Easy Fix: There is actually a science to making a smoothie really healthy and keeping you full. My smoothies always have a high quality protein powder, dark leafy greens, carbs and good fats. This combination helps balance the blood sugar and keeps you fuller for longer. My favourite is spinach, a good vanilla protein powder, unsweetened coconut milk, cacao powder (not to be confused with cocoa or chocolate), almond butter (without added sugar) and a banana. You have an easy, delicious, fat-blasting breakfast in minutes that keeps you full for hours. In the recipe section of this book we provide more detail and reveal the step-by-step guide to making a healthy and filling smoothie.

2. Choosing the wrong protein powder to add to your smoothie.

Mistake: Among a growing array of choices, finding the right protein powder can become a challenge. If you don't believe me, visit your local supermarket or health food store and read those labels. We discovered this in the previous section.

Easy Fix: choose non-soy, non-dairy protein powder. My favourite plant proteins include pea and hemp and proteins.

3. Turning your smoothie into a milkshake (that brings all the boys to the yard).

Mistake: I used to top up all my shakes with cow's milk and wondered why I was always bloated, spotty and wasn't losing weight even though I was replacing breakfast with a smoothie. Lactose is found in all dairy products and is a form of sugar. The sugar content in dairy is not off the scale high but it's enough to elevate your blood sugar levels, which can contribute to weight gain! Consequently, cutting back on dairy products can accelerate weightloss. This applies especially to dairy products that are lacking in fat, such as regular milk and low fat and diet yogurts as we uncovered earlier.

Most people do not produce enough of the digestive enzyme called lactase, which is responsible for effectively digesting lactose. This means a large number of the population go completely unaware that dairy is causing unnecessary gut irritations, which also prevents weightloss and increases other health issues, not to mention some embarrassing trips to the public loo.

Easy Fix: If you want a milky smoothie, choose a non-soy, non-dairy milk such as coconut, almond, hazelnut or hemp. Try them all and see which one you like best! Whichever you choose, make sure you get the UNSWEETENED version. The 'ORIGINAL' versions will be full of secret added sugars!

4. Buying powders and supplements with unhealthy toxic ingredients to add to your smoothie (for example, green powders or protein powders).

Mistake: Manufacturers make powders taste good with preservatives, maltodextrin, bulk fillers, artificial additives or flavorings and E-Numbers. They use tonnes of added sugar, such as fructose, corn syrup, other syrup, sugar alcohols, juice, concentrate, fructose and sweeteners. Those should all be red flags to put that powder back on the shelf or in the bin!

Natural sugar is different and includes sugar cane, coconut sugar or stevia leaf. The ones to watch out for are the processed and artificial sugars. Also, watch out for the online sales people selling these 'magic' products; their company's powders, pills and supplements. They are usually untrained in ingredients and nutrition and their main focus is to sell, not your health.

Easy Fix: Make sure you READ YOUR LABELS. Knowledge is power and simply because the advert or the label says it is good for you, doesn't mean it actually is!

It is up to you as an individual to check it out for yourself. Learn what these toxic ingredients are so you are fully aware of what you are putting into your body. Once you have looked into it, you can make a fully educated decision about whether you want to keep using it and my bet is when you know what you are putting into your body, you will want a better quality powder free of these toxic ingredients! This includes all processed food in the 'healthy' section of the supermarket. They are usually not what they seem. Make label reading a new hobby.

5. Using fruit juice as the liquid base to your smoothie.

Mistake: Fruit juice is often perceived as healthy...it's made from fruit, right?

Well, not always. Store bought juices are often actually not much more than fruit flavoured sugar water. In some cases, there may not even be any actual fruit in there...it may simply be water, sugar and additives that taste like fruit.

The problem with most high street fruit juice is that it's like fruit, except with all of the good bits taken out. To make fruit juice, firstly you have to remove all the fibre and then most juices available in regular supermarkets are pasturised. This means they have been heated during the manufacturing process, which is needed to prolong the shelf life. If we were to make fruit juice at home with a juicer, that juice would last between 24 – 48 hours before it goes off, so the pasteurisation is needed for juices to be sold in shops. However, when the fruit is heated, it loses almost all of its original nutrients and many top brands have to add synthetic vitamins to replace what has been lost. What you are left with is basically sugary water plus any other chemical additives. The sugar content of some store bought fruit juice is actually very similar to sugar sweetened fizzy beverages. Now some people have been told that all fruit is bad and to avoid it all, but this is a mistake. Fruit is great! Yes, whole fruits also contain sugar, but it is contained within its fibrous cell walls, which slows down the release of the sugar into the bloodstream. Fruit is FULL of vital vitamins and minerals we need. Nothing wrong with eating fruit! Some people worry about eating too much of it but it would be very difficult for a person to over eat on fruit.

Even IF you can get your hands on real, 100% cold pressed fruit juice, you still shouldn't be drinking that much of it. No more than one glass a day and preferably not in your morning weightloss smoothie as it has had its fibre removed.

Easy Fix: You are better off making your smoothie with water or non-dairy milk. If you want a fruity flavoured smoothie, blend **real** fruit into your shake rather than using juice. The sugar in whole fruit is unlike any other sugar available, plus it still has all its nutrients, which we need for good health. When we eat whole fruit, our body knows exactly how to use it as an energy source and we should never be scared to eat real whole fruits and veggies.

Smoothies for weightloss is a serious business!

I used to throw anything I could into the blender and press GO! I stopped losing weight, I put on weight and I felt hungry all the time, which made me reach for sugary snacks mid-morning before lunch. The right shake will make all the difference to your weightloss journey. Make it your mission to get it right!

MYTH – You think finding the next 'new' thing will be the answer to your prayers.

TRUTH – The truth is there is only ever ONE thing that will get you the permanent weightloss results. The ONLY thing that will get you LONG-TERM PERMENANT RESULTS is to PERMENANTLY CHANGE YOUR LIFESTYLE!

There is no single diet, new or old that will be the answer to your prayers. We need to stop searching and looking for the next new thing; the next shake; the next pill; the next supplement; the next challenge; the next way to starve and make ourselves miserable. That stuff simply doesn't work long term for most people. There are a few things you can do to start seeing the results you want. Firstly, decide to get serious and take a serious look at what you feed yourself on a daily basis and ask yourself, "Is it really good enough?" Secondly, understand that you might not be able to do this alone. Most people need a coach or someone to guide them and cheer them on. Thirdly, commit to loving yourself so much that only the best will do! Start making those healthy day-to-day choices and little by little you will start to get results. You could look at your shopping basket a year from today and barely recognise it. I still do that now! As I unpack my weekly shop, I simply cannot believe that it is truly MY shopping. Did I accidently grab someone else's trolley at check out? Did a magical elf somehow swap my shopping bags? My cupboards and fridge are full of colourful fruit and veg. Pulses. Nuts. Legumes. So much fresh food and not a package meal in sight! I used to live on my packaged low calorie meals and loved it...but I never understood my lack of energy. Well, not anymore! I am not on a diet, it is my lifestyle and I live it with ease without thinking about it. I am full of energy. It isn't an effort. It isn't complicated and I don't have to count numbers. Sometimes I will have a moment, a little wobble and go looking for junk in the kitchen. I will open the fridge and search, check the back of the cupboards and then, I remember I have no junk in the house because I don't need it any more. Instead, I have a little chat with myself, accept there is nothing 'rubbish' in my house anymore and I whip up a healthy alternative and I am good to go. This is because I stopped looking for the next best thing and simply started to change my life...one step at a time. Sometimes this is the hardest part. Know that this change is forever and this is the only way you are going to get the body of your dreams. How do we expect to lose weight and keep it off eating junk food 3 or 4 times a week and drinking diet fizzy drinks with meals. It is not gonna happen that way. We have to be honest about that.

If you want permanent change, **you** have to change **permanently**. It isn't easy and that is why I always recommend seeking a coach to lean on. You have to address lifelong habits and beliefs, which can be disheartening at times. But if I can do it, a lifelong sugar addict, then so can you. It was hard. I still fall back sometimes when I am stressed out, but because I have changed my lifestyle, I will never go back to the way I was before. I have to confess I spent a few months swimming in sugar recently. When my mum suddenly passed away, the only thing that would make me feel a teeny tiny bit better was chocolate, sweets and cake – and A LOT of it! It was hard and I nearly lost myself, but because I had started to do it right many years before by changing my lifestyle and dealing with my emotional eating, I was able to bring myself back again. I could no longer see my clients because I wasn't in the right headspace. The whole experience was very traumatic. My Mum was also a public figure, which meant I kept seeing her in the press and I was getting messages from all over the place. I simply wanted to hide away and eat, but I found other things to keep me occupied and focused because that was the only way to bring myself out of it. I handled it by writing this book. I had so much to share with other people and while I had to defer all my clients to my husband Josh, that didn't stop me from releasing my knowledge in this book for you and other women like you. Writing this stopped me from eating myself into a hole. It was hard. It still is hard when I think of her, but I refuse to go back, because I know I can find healthier alternatives and other things to keep me pushing forwards. This is why it is so important to find things other than food that make you feel good and this is the difference between the next 'new diet' and a permanent change in your life. Your new lifestyle becomes so normal to you that when you hit a roadblock and slip back to the way you were before, it will feel uncomfortable. It will feel so wrong that you want to get back to being better more than anything else in the world. You love yourself so much that only the best will do! If I managed to bring myself back from my shock and grief, I know you can too.

MYTH – You think weightloss is all about **looking** a certain way.

TRUTH – Yes, of course there is no denying it, we want to look good and feel hot when we look in the mirror or walk past a shop window. That feeling of slipping on those skinny jeans you hid at the back of the wardrobe is amazing. I know it all too well. But there is something that is much more important than how we look. And that is our health. Sometimes we get so caught up in how we look and what size jeans we are wearing, we forget the most important aspect, which is the overall level of our health. Ask yourself, is being skinnier more important than living a long and healthy life? Okay great we can see your rib cage, 'whoopdie do.' Being slim doesn't equal being healthy, looking good is only scratching the surface and actually isn't always enough to motivate us into sticking to our plan. Even when we know we are overweight and have too many wobbly bits, we sometimes get used it. It is comfortable. We buy the 'suck 'em in pants' and get on with it. I know. I used to too. We buy baggy tops and flowery peplum dresses to hide the bits we don't like. I know because I've done it! There are all sorts of tricks we can do to hide the fact that we aren't in great shape. But there is nothing out there in the market that will hide diabetes; or heart disease; or a stroke; or cancer. When we eat unhealthily, regardless of our size, we increase the risk of fatal diseases. Society is so focused on body image and body shaming that we have forgotten the most important reason to change our lifestyle and make healthier choices. This is another reason why I can't stand those faddy diets and weightloss clubs. Even if you lose weight on the diet in the club, none of those methods are healthy. You can be in skinny jeans and still at a high risk of heart disease or have high cholesterol. All the processed ready meals, diet foods and meal replacement shakes simply do not contain the nutrients our body needs to perform at its best. But we get so caught up on weigh-in day when we get a gold star or a certificate that we don't think of what the cost is to our health. This is why it is so important to do this properly. Not as fast as we can. Not in competition with any one, but by focusing on our lifelong journey to better our health.

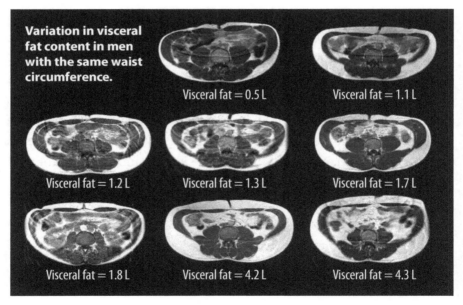

(Source: www.commons.wikimedia.org)

These are images of someone with the **same** waist measurements on the outside. They are likely to all be the same or similar clothes size too. However, when we look at what's inside; it is a very different story. The L numbers underneath each image tells us the amount of visceral fat, which is the fat on the **inside** of our body. Visceral fat that will be around our organs and our brain and can be inside of us regardless of what we look like on the outside. It will cause health problems. It will give you sore joints and inflammation. It will zap your energy. It will affect your sleep. It will reduce our immunity to the common cold and flu. It wreaks havoc inside us and is caused by an unhealthy lifestyle... again this includes people of all shapes and sizes both large and small. Take a second and think about your children or future children or your grandchildren. Do you want to be around for a long time and in good health for your family? Do you want to be able to run around or get up the stairs without getting out of breath? Then it is time to stop focusing on what you look like and actually look at what's beneath your skin. Are you thinking about your health long term or are you willing to do any unhealthy method just so you can look certain way?

I was fat-skinny for many years. That is what I call it, skinny looking on the outside but full of visceral fat on the inside. I slimmed to a size 6 – 8, I thought I looked great, but was still eating highly processed foods, too much meat and dairy and having a lot of sugary foods. I had managed to keep my body shape pretty good by being very active and dancing an awful lot. I was working in Disneyland Paris as a dancer and character performer, which was much like working out 24/7. But when I checked my visceral fat, it was awful! I was shocked at what I was doing to my body while kidding myself that it was okay because I was a size 8. I had to look a little deeper and get real with myself. I decided to clean up my act and started to make healthy choices. I had more energy, my skin cleared up, I lost the fluffy bit round the middle and I felt great! Have a talk with yourself today. Are you doing this for the skinny jeans or good health? It can be a bit of both of course, but remember to always put your health first. Losing weight doesn't mean you are healthy, where as being healthy almost always guarantees fat loss will follow naturally. We have gotten it wrong for so many years. It is time to get it right. Focus on being healthy **first**; eating **real** food; less processed foods; and more fruit and veggies; and pack in those nutrients rather than focusing on weightloss foods or low fat or diet foods. Weightloss and losing weight any old way doesn't always mean you are strong and healthy, but being healthy and making healthier food decisions almost always leads to fat loss and weightloss. Make sense?

There is a lot to take in. But the moral of the story is this; HEALTH over weightloss any day. We have to start using our common sense and question what we currently know.

CHAPTER 4: Mindset

Most people think weightloss is all about food and willpower. While it is true you need an element of willpower and yes you need to eat the right foods, the success of your journey is not all about food and willpower. You can have as many food lists as you like, join every diet club and sign up to every gym in town. Until you get your MINDSET in check, you will ALWAYS slip back into old habits eventually.

What do we mean when we say mindset? Well it can mean many things. We focus on this in our programs, but for the purpose of this book, let's talk about two things to get our juices flowing.

The first thing in the area of mindset to talk about is how you feel about yourself and the love you have for yourself. Self-loving plays a role in long-term weightloss and health and is often forgotten. If you label yourself 'fat', feel like you aren't good enough and feel worthless, you are more likely to find it harder to make healthier food choices when left to your own devices, because deep down you believe you are fat, therefore you make 'fat choices'. You will be okay with feeding yourself Maccy Ds. You will feel okay with eating the processed ready meals. You will feel okay with not eating enough nutrients. This is because deep down you haven't realised yet that you deserve better. Now don't get me wrong, I am not saying I am perfect and yes, I still hate my hips sometimes, but most of the time I simply love myself too much to continually feed my body rubbish. I do like Maccy Ds but when I think about eating it I know I couldn't bring myself to do it. It's not even real food really is it? I simply love myself enough to want to give my body the best fuel. This wasn't an overnight thing. This is something that can take time and we work with our clients to help them on this self-love journey, but when you have true love for yourself, you simply will not want to keep giving yourself junk all the time. You will respect your body so much that you simply rise above the junk because it isn't good enough for you. It won't be so hard to say no to the biscuits that get passed round every day at work and it will be easy to drink a green smoothie for breakfast instead of a grabbing a muffin at the corner shop on the way to work.

Depending on where you are in your journey right now, you might think this is a bit farfetched and those of you who have had a glimpse of real self-love will know exactly what I am talking about. For those of you who aren't quite there yet, I urge you to keep going. Humour me and give this a go. Start telling yourself you love yourself. Tell yourself that you are enough as you are. Stop labelling yourself fat. YOU aren't fat. Nobody IS fat. We might HAVE fat on us yes, but we aren't all fat. Stop giving yourself this derogatory label. The fat on your body doesn't, nor will it ever define WHO you are. You HAVE fat like you HAVE fingers or toes. While we need and want our fingers and toes, we might not want the fat, but calling ourselves fat makes us feel crappy. It encourages you to make bad decisions, which in turn, takes you further away from your goal of getting rid of the extra fat. Instead, be okay with being on this journey, don't beat yourself up about it, embrace it and embrace yourself. The more self-love you have, the easier it will become to make healthier decisions and say no to junk. It is all in the mindset and the wording. You aren't fat. You are simply working on getting rid of some of the excess fat that your body doesn't need.

The second part of mindset I want to talk about in this book is our emotional foodie crutches. That's my personal term for the food we turn to when we feel bad to make us feel better. Our foodie crutches are how we suppress our true feelings. Instead of facing our feelings head on, we lean on certain foods as a way of dealing with our problems. Emotional eating is all about our mindset and addressing our true feelings. Society has most of us believing that it isn't okay to not be okay. We have somehow started to believe we should suppress our emotions and instead of facing problems head on, we hide behind food (or alcohol) to make us feel better. We see it on television and movies all the time. Guy dumps the girl, so the girlfriends binge on ice cream to make them feel happy again.

Most of us learn that **food/eating = happiness** from our parents and society, but we usually have no idea we are doing it until we start to feel out of control. The trouble is once we have used our foodie crutch, the problem we had to start with is usually still there and we beat ourselves up for bingeing or pigging out. The foodie crutch gives us short-term relief followed by longer-term guilt.

The first step to winning this war on emotional eating is to open your eyes about the fact you are doing it in the first place. When we live in denial, we will never gain back the control. But by being real with ourselves and putting our hands up and admitting it, we will start to understand our patterns and find ways of overcoming it.

"Hi! I am Ahisha and I am an emotional eater."

Sounds cheesy, I know, but if you can't admit this, you have already lost the war. Yes, it is a war; a battle to fight against all those life-long habits we have been taught; a combat against the fake beliefs that we think are fact. Eventually, we can start to separate the feelings of emotions we have connected to the food we eat. We will still enjoy food, but we will no longer eat mindlessly and feel out of control. We will eat those foods because we choose to – cheat meal – but not because we feel we **have** to. We will see food for what it truly is – fuel – and we will find our happiness elsewhere. We will learn how to feel our emotions instead of suppressing them with cake. We will explore how we feel and find other ways to clear our minds and deal with our problems. But before that happens, we must first assess the situation. We must open our eyes.

Here is another task we set for our clients who struggle with understanding their habits and mindset.

This series of questions will help to uncover your story so you can start to take back control. If you have the physical book, grab a pen and write notes in the boxes and answer the questions. Or if you have a digital copy grab a notebook. However you decide to do it, please just do it. Most people surprise themselves with the answers.

Question #1

What do you think your emotional foodie crutches are and where/how do you think it started?

TIP: Have a think about the foods you crave when you are feeling down, stressed, upset. Did you see your parents do this? Was it after an emotional period in your life?

_____

_____

_____

_____

Question #2

What usually triggers you to reach for these foods?

TIP: Think about WHY you feel upset at these times, for example, a long day at work, arguing with your partner or loneliness etc.

_____

_____

_____

_____

Question #3

How does it make you feel when you eat these foods?

TIP: Think about how you feel before, during and after a 'bingeing' session.

_____

_____

_____

_____

Question #4

What practical tools can you start to put in place to begin the process of disconnecting the emotion you have tied to it?

TIP: Can you remove the triggers from your life? Can you swap the junk for healthier alternatives? Can you talk about a problem with someone? Could you use your list of things that make you happy?

_____

_____

_____

_____

While weightloss is about the food we eat and having an element of willpower, the biggest success will be celebrated once you break free of your emotional eating and get your mindset in check. Most diet clubs or weightloss programs simply do not address these every day struggles we face, which is why they are set up to make you feel a failure. It's not you. It's them.

For most people, this task of exploring emotional eating can be difficult. It can be painful sometimes as you are forced to think deeper. Don't hide from it, don't be afraid to look inside yourself and try a new approach. If in doubt, my details are at the back, drop me an email and we can explore this together.

Ultimately, this is your journey of self-discovery. You can start to finally uncover and understand why you do the things you do. Why you eat the way you do? Why do some days feel harder to stick to the plan than other days? The more you understand yourself, the less you will blame yourself for you mistakes.

CHAPTER 5:

Change Your Weightloss Approach

If we carry on with the current approach to weight loss, we will carry on being unhappy, hungry and frustrated. Why continue doing something that isn't serving you? It is time to switch it up a bit, change our approach to achieve the results we are searching for. Here are some top tips to get you started.

Read your labels!

When food has green packaging and the advert says it is **healthy**, it doesn't actually mean that it is. The government guidelines on what is classed as 'healthy' are blurred and these guidelines change on a yearly basis. We must start to read the labels to understand what is actually **inside** the products we are buying. Knowledge is power and we need to know what we are putting in our body, not only what the advert tells us. A product in a green package with the word 'healthy' written on it doesn't mean that it is all natural and good for you. It's simply clever marketing and branding. Turn the package over and have a proper look.

Put your health before your weightloss

This might sound crazy but it truly makes perfect sense. Here is a quote we made up for our clients

"Once you get your nutrition right, that's when the magic will happen."

What you look like on the outside will change when you focus on feeding the best stuff to the inside. This means no more looking for quick fix diet pills, starving and fasting or diet foods. This is all about putting more **nutrient dense** food into your body and giving it the best fuel you can possibly find.

Work on YOU!

Getting to work on **you** is going to make this journey much easier. Accept that you need to address your old habits and old lifestyle and start to embrace the fact that if you want change in your life, YOU will have to change. You simply cannot expect to stay the same while everything else changes. This will leave you feeling frustrated and resentful every time. You have to get real and give yourself a talking to if you want long-term weightloss. Many times before we speak to a client they are adamant that they are healthy enough already, but when we look at their food diary it turns out they could be eating half a pack of biscuits every day and totally unaware of it. A biscuit here and there is so easy to overlook because it becomes a (mindless) habit. It is usually a similar story: the office worker has 2 biscuits when the pack is passed around for elevenses. Then another 2 or 3 when it is passed round later in the afternoon. You get home and grab a biscuit while you prepare the dinner and then you have another 3 when you are settling in for an evening of 'soaps' on the television. It doesn't seem like a lot but they add up over a day and a week. Unless you start to take notice of your daily habits and lifestyle, you will always wonder where you are going wrong when the answer might be right under your own nose. It is time to wake up your sub-conscious mind and start to look consciously and mindfully at what you eat.

Stop beating yourself up!

Guess what? This is not gonna be easy. Changing any lifelong habit is hard work and the sooner you admit this, the faster you can stop being so darn hard on yourself! Yes, you need to be real with yourself and honest with what you are **really** eating, but once you have done that and start to make changes don't be hard on yourself when you slip up. Slipping up doesn't make you a failure. Slipping up makes you **human**! When you do slip up and lose track, it is important to admit it, but don't dwell on it, don't beat yourself up and certainly don't give up because you had a minor slip up. You know that feeling where you were doing so well but then slipped up with that slice of cake at the work party? Or the feeling after you ate those biscuits after a stressed week, it was meant to be one biscuit but somehow the pack accidently finished? Then when you sit and say to yourself, 'Well, I had that slice of cake/pack of biscuits earlier, I may as well have the crisps in the cupboard now.' The next morning you feel bad. You feel like you messed up so bad and you punish yourself by branding yourself a failure and stop at the bakery on the way to work. You are off the wagon now, may as well carry on. That weekend you grab a Maccy Ds and have a few glasses of wine with the girls and before you know it, you are so far away from your track you can't even see the wood though the trees. You look around and you are surrounded by all your old habits again and wonder how you got there. What comes next? Even more punishment, where you decide to give up cake for the rest of your life, start working out like a mad woman and start eating salad every day. (BORING! How many people actually love salad that much?) This type of thinking never lasts and you are torturing yourself. All because you had that one slice of cake or those biscuits!

Do yourself a massive a favour. The next time you slip up and have the cake at the work party, simply stop there. One slip up isn't the end of the world. You don't need to dwell on it and spiral out of control. Stop blowing these little things out of proportion. Yes, it is important to be real about it. Don't pretend like it didn't happen. Acknowledge it and accept you slipped up, learn from it and move on! We all slip up. I still slip even now...but I know that a piece of cake is simply a piece of cake. It doesn't mean I am a failure and it doesn't mean I should spiral out of control and eat everything else I see in front of me for the next week, or starve myself as punishment. It is okay to make mistakes. When we beat ourselves up and tell our self how bad we are and how we've got no willpower, we are sabotaging our self and delaying our own success. Saying, "Oh, I've had a piece of cake I may as well give up for the week and start again on Monday," is quite simply crazy. Sorry, but it is! One mistake doesn't mean you need to give up and start again the next week. It means do your best for the rest of the week to stick to your plan. If your car had one flat tyre would you slash all the other three to match? No! You would simply fix the ONE that was bad and keep on along your journey. Stop slashing all your tyres! We aren't perfect. This won't be a perfect journey. But this will be your **journey** and it will be amazing! But you must stop striving for perfection and be okay with making a few mistakes.

Okay, so what next? We have come to the end of the 3 Key Secrets that you need to know. We've done the first steps of uncovering some huge myths and replacing them with real truths and we've started looking at ways to change your approach, but what now? Now we are going to start on the next part of revealing the formula you need to move forward. The formula you need to ensure you get the success you deserve. The formula we share with all our clients to help them finally lose weight and keep it off for good without dieting or starving or counting calories. It is a 6 step formula and you will be happy to know we have already started uncovering the first 5 steps.

What have we discovered so far?

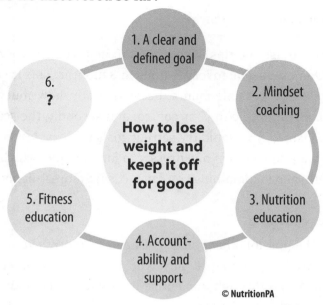

© NutritionPA

1. A clear and defined goal

No goal means you will never be able to track any sort of success. A goal helps you get organised and plan out your day-to-day. It helps you celebrate your success and keeps you focused. When we get into a car we turn on the sat nav and put in the destination so we know where we are going. It wouldn't make sense to turn on the sat nav and not enter the location address, would it? You would end up driving around in circles and never reach your destination. The same goes for anything we want to achieve in life. When we have put in that destination and set our plan, it gives us something to follow. Even when we go off track, or take a detour, the sat nav will always get us to the destination in the end.

Factors to think about when setting your goal

- What is your goal?
- How is it measured?

- How will you know when you reach it?
- Is your goal measured fairly?

Make sure you use the tips in this book to help you set your goal. For example, don't set a goal to lose 5 stone in 3 months. This is setting you up for stress and possible failure, because firstly, how much you lose and when, might not be in your control and secondly, the scales might lie to you. Instead, you could try setting goals such as; I won't skip any meals; or I aim to go down one dress size for example, which gives you more control and is something you can measure more reliably and fairly.

2. Mindset coaching

Accepting the possibly that you might need to address your emotional eating, as well as looking at how you feel about yourself is really important. We go through our entire lives with these bad habits and being emotionally attached to our food. Most of the time willpower isn't enough to break through this lifetime of bad habit. Discovering how to deal with our emotional eating is a key step in moving forward and never having to diet again.

3. Nutrition education

Learning about food and your body really gives you the upper hand when it comes to making healthier choices. Understanding how your body processes what you feed it will help you feel more in control. Understanding what the consequences of eating junk food are can make such a difference to your journey.

We all already knew that sugar was bad for us, but how do you feel now you know about the blood sugar balance and how blood sugar spikes lead to crashing and more sugary cravings?

- Now you know the logical reasoning behind what snacks to choose, will it make you think twice before choosing your next snack?

- Now you know that your body goes into starvation mode when you skip meals, will you start to make more of an effort to eat your meals instead of going hungry?
- Now you know that diet foods are full of rubbish, are you more likely to check the ingredients next time you are at the supermarket?

Most of you will answer, yes, yes and yes!

Our choices become less about willpower and more about us genuinely wanting to stop treating our body badly. Knowledge really is power and the more you know about food, nutrition and your body, the better decisions you start to make and the easier it will be to lose weight and keep it off for good.

4. Accountability and support

Why try and figure it all out on your own when you can have the support of a coach to lead you all the way to the finish line and to help set goals? To help answer all those tricky nutrition questions. To help boost you when you are feeling down and to stop you spiraling out of control when you hit a rough patch. To help keep you motivated so you stick to your goals. To help you work through any emotional eating or mindset road clocks. To ground you and keep you sane! This journey isn't easy, but it needn't be so hard either and you can take a load off simply by having a Nutrition and Health Coach. People are so quick to get themselves a Personal Trainer for their fitness but who is taking care of the nutritional side? In the United States, it is a lot more common, but not so much in the United Kingdom. My husband and I are coaches as well as nutritional therapists and even we need support along our own journey. My husband Josh has Sickle Cell disease and his requirements are very specific. He needs guidance from specialists from time to time. I am a self-confessed sugar addict and emotional eater and I need someone to whip me into shape and give me a kick up the bum at times. Yes, I know all the nutrition stuff, but I need someone to get me out of my own way and keep me on track. It is all too easy to fall into old habits and not notice. My husband is my guide. He is the first one to pull me up and say "But didn't you already have your cheat meal this week?" Yes, it is frustrating to be pulled up on little mistakes but in the end, I am really grateful to have someone looking out for me who has got my back. As nutrition coaches we are always here to support our clients and hold them accountable for their individual goals. We are the 'Nutrition PAs', the personal assistants in all things health and food related. My favourite part of the job is when we reach a goal with a client and we celebrate and congratulate them for their work. Seeing the journey unfold fills my heart with such joy and happiness.

5. Fitness education

Similar to nutrition education, understand how to properly exercise. Finding what exactly you enjoy can make all the difference between actually doing it or not. Instead of simply going to the gym and forcing yourself to do what you think you should be doing, you can actually find something you enjoy and stick to it. How different will it feel knowing you can achieve your goal through a really fun fitness class rather than running on a boring treadmill? Well, this is assuming that like me you don't like the treadmill! What a weight lifted off my shoulders – and my wallet – when I found out I didn't have to go to the gym anymore and I could still achieve my goals in other ways. Maybe it is time to try classes or speak to different instructors for advice. There are so many ways to keep fit, go out and have fun experimenting.

6. What is the sixth key to our success formula that we haven't looked at yet? This maybe is the most important thing to know **before** embarking on any new lifestyle change. This is the step that makes most of our clients scared and excited at the same time. Let's explore the sixth key to success. Long-term dieting has left our body and minds in such a mess quite frankly, so changing our lifestyle on top of all the bad habits can be quite challenging and overwhelming. It is like when you try to paint a fresh layer of nail polish on the old chipped layer underneath. While the new colour will fill the gaps, the end result is uneven and bumpy. Some of the old colour from underneath might even show through in parts. Not the look we are trying to achieve is it? The same happens when we try and create new habits ON TOP of old ones. It can get cloudy and confusing. Our body and mind doesn't know what to do or where to start sometimes. We will have the same old cravings and the same old habits holding us back and getting in the way. But what if we can wipe the slate clean? What if we can remove cravings or at least reduce them? Wouldn't it be better if we were to build a new lifestyle from scratch? Get rid of the old and start something new? Well, there is a way. This is the first step on our client program and it is called The Detox Without Deprivation. Let's take a closer look!

CHAPTER 6:

The Detox Without Deprivation

Why detox?

Firstly, before you think I have lost the plot, I want to share why detoxing should always be the first step to creating a new lifestyle. Some people do not believe in detoxing and think there is no need for it because our body detoxes itself, which it does to a point. Well, I am here to say that there is 100% a need for it, but not any old detox...a very special type of detox, which I will feature shortly.

Think about it. It is the 21st century and we live in a toxic world. We only need to trace our steps for a day and see what toxins our body is bombarded with on a daily basis.

We get up and get ready to go out. Toothpaste, shower gel, soap, make up all contain hundreds of ingredients, which are toxic to us. Did you know that what we put on our skin sinks into our blood stream? Before we leave the house we could have easily chucked on an average 500+ chemicals into our blood stream already. The foods we eat are full of additives, preservatives, antibiotics, pesticides and more, unless you already eat 100% organic and non-GMO foods. The air we breathe, especially in cities, is smoggy and full of dust and fumes.

We are living in a toxic world. I hear what you are thinking, "Of course, I cannot stay indoors and avoid this. I have to live, don't I?"

But at the same time we are filling our bodies with toxins. These toxins are one of the biggest contributing factors to why we are getting sicker and gaining more fat as a population, although we are a more health conscious society than ever before. How can that be; more health conscious but getting sicker? The problem is toxic overload. That is why detoxing will always be useful, especially for weightloss!

"But surely our bodies can handle it or we would all be dead?"

That is a question I hear quite often. Well, day-to-day toxins will not kill you on the spot now, but toxic overload in our bodies will reduce our immune system and zap our energy.

The main job of our liver is to get rid of these foreign toxic particles in our body, but as time has gone on, we are ingesting more toxins and our livers are over worked and over tired. Detoxing is about giving our liver a break and a chance to get rid of excess toxins that have built up in our bodies.

Here is an example, which I heard from another wonderful nutritional expert.

Imagine you work at airport security and it is your job to check all the hand luggage bags. You have to be awake and fully functioning to view thousands of bags each day for dangerous items. Knives, guns, suspicious powders and of course, any liquids contained in a bottle bigger than 100ml! As part of your job at security, you get a lunch break, a tea break, you go home to your family every day at 5pm to relax and sleep 8 hours at night before coming in to work again the next day. You eat, you sleep and you hydrate so your job can be done effectively. In addition, twice a year you go on holiday. All is good until one day your boss comes in and tells you your contract has changed. You no longer get breaks on shift. You now work 24 hours a day, 7 days a week, with no breaks or holiday time! Obviously, this is illegal, but if it weren't – let's pretend for the sake of making a point – what do you think would happen to the quality of your work if you never had a break? You would start to get tired wouldn't you? You would get sloppy and unfocused and ultimately, you would start to let dangerous items through because you wouldn't be able to do your job effectively.

This is the life of your liver.

It is working to expel harmful toxins from your body day and night. While you sit there right now reading this book, your liver is hard at work; like your ears, lungs and brains. Our body never stops working. Take a moment and think about that for a second. You are swallowing every so often and your eyelids are blinking every 4 seconds on average and you didn't even realize it! Until I pointed it out that is. You are probably aware of your eyes blinking and your bodily functions right now more in this very moment than you have been before. It's amazing isn't it? How your body simply does its thing. It is like a machine; every part doing its bit to keep us alive; to keep us functioning. Our body works really hard for us, day in and day out.

Anyway, back to the liver. Toxins enter our body via 3 main routes, our skin, our lungs (when we breathe) and our guts. Yes, our guts! Did you know that the average person has between 6 – 20 pounds of undigested waste sitting in our intestines! Sitting there, rotting away? Guess what? If that food is a toxic food, such as hormone filled meat or processed chemical food, it is also leaching toxins into our bodies day in and day out, which our liver has to work at getting rid of as quickly and safely as possible. Our body gets rid of toxins in 4 ways. I call them the 4 Ps.

- Pee
- Poop

- Perspiration (sweat)
- Pranayama (breath)

Let's get into the science of how our body detoxes itself and how we can help it out a little.

The pee comes from our kidneys working for us. Help your kidneys by drinking plenty of water. Pee should be almost clear and odourless. If you have smelly yellow wee, your body is highly toxic and you are probably dehydrated too. Many people find drinking more water tricky, including me. We lead busy lives and drinking water can easily fall down the priority list. One tip that can help you as it did me is to download an App called Water Balance. This App has changed my water habits for life. It gives you a visual representation of what you are drinking long with little watery tips and facts along the way. It is free to download so give it a go.

The poop comes from our colon, which is the last place waste goes before we poop it out. This might be gross, but it's time to get dirty and talk about poop! Don't be shy now it is only you and me here, together. When was the last time you took notice of your poop? What does it look like? How often do you go? Poop is a huge indicator of how our digestive system is working and how effective we are at clearing what we eat out of our bodies. Did you know that technically we are meant to poop the same amount of times a day that we eat? Which means if we are eating 3 times a day, then really we should be pooping 3 times a day. Just like a baby. If you have ever been on nappy duty, you will know how many times we poop as babies.

My goodness, I felt like I was knee deep in poop when my son was a baby. This is when our digestive system is brand new. No backlog. No issues. Food comes in waste comes out; very simple. Not anymore! We are eating so many things that we shouldn't be eating and to top it off, not eating enough fibre that our digestive systems are suffering. We simply aren't pooping as much as we should. When I first moved in with Josh, one day he asked me, "Do you poo?"

I was confused why he was asking. "'Course, I poo!!" I replied.

"When did you last poo?" he said.

Then next came silence. Followed by tumbleweed. I couldn't answer him because I didn't know the last time I had pooed. I wasn't counting my poos, (what normal person counts their poos, right?) But also at that moment I realised that I was probably only pooing every other day! Gross! All that food was sitting there in my gut leaching out toxins and making me bloated and tired. Something to think about isn't it? Help our bodies remove toxic and rotting waste by again, drinking plenty of water and also making sure you get enough fibre. Most people on average in the United Kingdom eat about 18 grams of fibre per day, but really we should be eating no less than 30 grams for optimum digestive health. Help your poop to help your body detox via your colon.

Moving swiftly on from poop, I think you get the point.

Perspiration comes from our skin sweating out of our pores. We can help our body by working out and getting ourselves in a sweat. What sort of working out you do is totally up to you, but toxins come out in our sweat. You could even try a session in the sauna or steam room for those days when you have a headache or can't be bothered. The other way to help our bodies to sweat is by watching what we put on our skin. Our skin is our largest organ and one of its main jobs is to breathe and let out toxins, but certain chemicals stop it from doing its job effectively. Petroleum, petrolatum and mineral oil all stop our bodies from breathing and letting out toxins. It covers our skin like cling film and blocks our pores from breathing. Have a look at your current skin care products and make sure it doesn't contain those pore blocking ingredients and help your skin sweat more effectively.

Pranayama is our lungs; breathing. In our breath, we can let out toxins. A great way to help our bodies do this is via meditation, yoga or Tai Chi, which all focus on our breath and breathing deeply. Or even better, you can get chatty! I have this joke in my seminars where I say that I am detoxing while giving my talk because I am breathing a lot. It gets a few laughs, but if you aren't laughing right it's because it probably works better in person. Talking is a great way to get breath in and toxins out via our lungs.

Yes, our body has its own way of detoxing and we can certainly help our bodies do their thing naturally. BUT and that is a capital BUT, it can only get rid of so much and sometimes needs intervention and help to give it a boost. Many years ago our livers wouldn't have been under so much stress. The air was cleaner and food was cleaner, but because now we are living in more and more of a toxic world, our livers are struggling to keep up in its natural process.

How do we know we need to detox and help our livers?

Our body is clever. It can't talk to us so it sends us signs and signals when it needs something. We know when we are hungry for example, because our tummy will rumble. In that same way our body sends us signs when it is struggling with some sort of toxic overload or difficulty, sort of like sending an SOS. Let's look at the 4 main signs, which could mean your body is crying out for a detox. There are many signs, but these are the top 4 signs most people experience.

Signal number 1 is SKIN

Are you suffering from skin irritations or acne breakouts? This is our bodies' way of letting us know something is up on the inside. Our skin is almost like a window to the inside. People who are wheat intolerant for example, may get eczema or dry skin when they consume wheat because it is toxic to them. The eczema is a sign from the body to explain that wheat is a problem. Another common one are spots after eating dairy. How is your skin holding up?

Signal number 2 is ENERGY LEVELS

Are you always tired? Or perhaps you have energy dips in the middle of the day. A lack of energy is a clear signal from our body that it is being over worked and it needs a break. We get so used to feeling lethargic that we begin to believe its normal, but in reality it is not at all normal. Unless you are pregnant, have a chronic illness, are more than 65 years old or have screaming babies keeping you up all night; the truth is we shouldn't always be so tired. We should be full of life all day. I know you probably don't believe me but it is true. I used to crash every day at 4pm and need a coffee. This was part of my normal routine. It was so normal that I didn't think twice or even once about it. But then I did my first detox without deprivation and boy, oh boy, was I surprised to suddenly be a ball of fire. There is a saying that couldn't be truer. "You do not know how good our body is designed to feel." Until you experience it, you will never really know what I am on about, but when you do experience it, you will never want to go back to the way you were before, the way you are now. Being full of energy will be the **new** normal and you will love it!

Signal number 3 is SUGAR CRAVINGS

We all know sugar is bad. We know it stops weightloss. We know it is bad for our teeth. Some of us are now aware that sugar accelerates cancer cell growth too. Yet, even though we know this, we continue to eat it because our body has uncontrollable cravings! These cravings are a sign that we need to detox from sugar because our body is addictive and on a dangerous endless sugar cycle loop.

This is the never-ending cycle of sugar cravings and yes, another of my gorgeous diagrams for you!

1. You Eat Sugar
You like it. It tastes GOOD!

2. Blood sugar levels spike
Happy hormones released into the body which is what makes sugar so addictive.

3. Hunger and cravings kick in
Low blood sugar levels increase your appetite. Sugar cravings kick in with an urge to get back that happy hormone high.

4. Blood sugar levels fall rapidly
High insulin levels are released into the body to try and bring sugar levels back to a normal range, which also creates excess fat storage.

© NutritionPA

This was me; I was hooked and those sugar cravings wouldn't go away. I wasn't in control and it doesn't stop. It goes round and round, and round and round. I was on a sugar cycle loop and the **only** thing that worked to break this cycle was to detox from processed and refined sugars, which are addictive and dangerous. This was a big sign for me that something had to change. Again, I am not saying I'm perfect and especially around Christmas time, I find myself suddenly on this sugar loop again. But because I now recognise it and understand the symptoms and the scientific process about it, I can spot what is going on, which means I now find it easier to jump off the loop when the celebrations are finished.

Rather than what I used to do, which was carry on well into January February and March, which totally ruined any New Year's resolutions.

Signal number 4 is DIGESTIVE ISSUES

This can show up for people in many different ways, shapes and forms. But they are a sign that you are feeding your body something that it cannot deal with effectively. One of the best ways to ease this issue is to detox from the most common digestive irritants and then at a later date, add them back in one at a time very slowly and asses how you feel. This requires you to stop ignoring those pesky symptoms and listen to your body. Something most of us fail to do, myself included. I used to think it was totally normal to be bloated...all the time! I thought that was simply the way I was made. I didn't think it was possible for me to be unbloated. Little did I know it was a sign; a sign from my body that I was ignoring. Our bodies are talking to us every day and giving us the clues we need to help us feel better. All we have to do is stop and listen once. It is so easy to get used to the bloating after we eat pizza or pasta and easy to ignore that bout of diarrhea after our ice cream binge. Easy to run and hide when we are having a gassy day. We get used to reaching for the medicine for that heartburn. Easy to overlook that time we got constipation. We start to think Irritable Bowel Syndrome and Chrones disease are part of who we are. I am telling you now, none of that is normal and we shouldn't get used to it or overlook any of it. They are all signs from our body that the digestive system is over worked and inflamed and untimely, it needs a break! Detoxing is the perfect way to give it that break it deserves and needs.

I am yet to meet a person who doesn't have at least 1 of those 4 signs. Most people have 2 or 3 signs, some have 1, a few have all 4, but never have I seen a person with zero signs. We need to stop ignoring these signs and listen to our body. Give it what it needs, a break!

What happens to excess toxins that cannot be expelled quickly enough?

Well, quite frankly, the excess toxins from this new toxic world we live in that aren't expelled fast enough, end up being deposited in various places around our bodies. One of the most popular places for excess toxins to be stored is our fat cells. Excess toxins stored in a fat cell are safer than left flowing around our bodies via blood stream, which can cause us to become sick with diseases. I call excess fat the bubble wrap for toxins.

How can detoxing help us lose weight and keep it off?

By now you might be thinking, that's great to know, but how will this help with losing weight?

Here is the clever part that will connect detoxing to that permanent weightloss we desire.

Have you ever been working out or 'dieting' and all is going well until you randomly hit a brick wall and plateau. Where that stubborn bit round the middle or on the arms won't budge no matter what you do. Or when you have eventually reached your weightloss goal but then you start to pile the weight back on again, commonly known as the 'yo-yo'. Remember, this is not your fault. There is a science and reason behind this. Breathe a sigh of relief because it isn't you. Many people go through this pattern of behavior and you are not alone. One of the reasons we plateau or yo-yo is because we have excess toxins that can't be expelled fast enough.

And get this; our body is smart! It is clever and springs into action to save the day! Our body will simply not let go of those fat cells if they are being used to store excess toxins. Our bodies are trying to keep us alive and they know that toxins are better off in a nice bit of bubble wrap – a fat cell – rather than in our blood steam. It will only release those fat cells when our overall level of toxins in the body go down to a safe enough level that it can handle safely.

Let's break it down.

Every time we lose weight without detoxing first, our body will start to let go of the fat. As it does this, any excess toxins are released from their safe fatty bubbles and forced out into our blood stream, which can wreak havoc around our body. The liver goes into red alert mode to start getting rid of as many toxins as possible. If the liver cannot get rid of these toxins fast enough, your body will go into over drive creating **more fat** cells to capture these toxins again. Excess toxins are always safer in fat than swimming around our body. Your body will always have your best interests at heart and if you are too toxic, it will always work against your best weightloss efforts to keep you safe on the inside. Detoxing is the way forward to boost weightloss and help you keep it off for good. Fat will begin to melt away and lean muscle mass is gained. You will have a better overall health and vitality.

Let's have a look at another of my diagrams. Visuals always help me, I hope they help you too! You may have seen variations of this one elsewhere but I am sure you will agree mine is the best one (I think...I hope!).

But wait...

MYTH – You think detoxing means starving yourself and depriving yourself from all food or having to survive on weird rabbit type foods or juices.

TRUTH – Think again! Detoxing has been turned into another faddy diet and any detox that requires you to starve can be dangerous and counter-productive to your overall long-term goals. Did you know that you can detox your body while eating 3 meals a day and snacks in between if you are hungry? Praise the Lord! We can eat AND detox! Who wants to survive on 3 shakes or juices a day? Certainly not me, I need to eat! I love to eat! No joke, the idea of having to not eat fills me with horror.

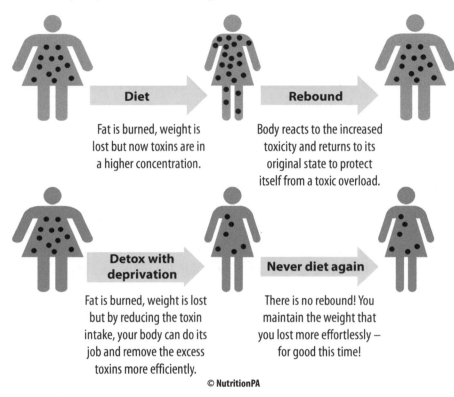

Diet

Fat is burned, weight is lost but now toxins are in a higher concentration.

Rebound

Body reacts to the increased toxicity and returns to its original state to protect itself from a toxic overload.

Detox with deprivation

Fat is burned, weight is lost but by reducing the toxin intake, your body can do its job and remove the excess toxins more efficiently.

Never diet again

There is no rebound! You maintain the weight that you lost more effortlessly – for good this time!

© NutritionPA

The truth is, when you deprive your body of the critical vitamins, minerals, proteins, fibres and carbohydrates it **needs**, you will suffer long term. Most mainstream 'detoxes' are just another form of quick fix dieting and teaches us nothing about your permanent lifestyle changes. Fasting is acceptable if you do it for religious reasons, but it isn't a good practice for weightloss. You will have cravings and be starving hungry. You may lose weight while not eating, but you will put it back on again when you start eating again. The same goes for the tea drinking, the juices and homemade shake detoxes. While these can be beneficial in some ways, they fail to address long-term habits and when you go back to the normal **old** lifestyle, you will put back on any weight you lost before and then some! So, what can we do?

We can detox **without** depriving ourselves of food!

In short, this means removing as many toxins as we possibly can at the same time as flooding our body with nutrient dense food to enhance our natural detoxing functions. This simultaneous act will help boost weightloss, start to heal our gut, boost our immune system and reduce cravings for junk food. As we flood ourselves with the good stuff, our body will start to crave more good stuff. It starts to change our taste buds and when we try to go back to the way we were before, we simply don't have the same taste for it as we once did. I used to LOVE Ribena and I was obsessed with that berry goodness. But now it tastes awful and more like sugary water. It certainly does not taste of berries anymore! I can't believe I used to think it actually tasted like fruit! Most cakes taste too sweet for me too. I have 1 slice and I am done, whereas before I could want more even after 4 slices! My taste buds were used to artificial rubbish, but not anymore, thanks to detoxing without depriving myself and flooding my body with the good stuff. The funny thing is, your body will always crave more of what you feed it. When you are feeding yourself artificial processed or sugary foods that is exactly what it will crave more of. If you feed your body green smoothies, guess what? It will start to crave more of those green smoothies.

Again, there is plenty of science to back this up. Our body actually renews and regenerates repetitively, day after day, year after year. Our skin regenerates every 4 to 6 weeks. As we get older, this process slows down, which is why as we age we lose that youthful glow, because our skin takes longer to renew. Your fingernails take 6 to 10 months to renew. I used to have such weak and brittle nails when my diet was full of junk. Now I eat so many legumes and pulses, which are high in calcium, my nails are AMAZING! I feel like I am wearing fake nails now in comparison. It took time, but they are not the same nails they were before. I sometimes sit and stare at them…even Josh gives them a little stroke every now and then! Ha ha! Taste buds renew themselves, the lungs, red blood cells and our hair! Our body is constantly rebuilding and growing. Each day is a new day for you to literally **rebuild** a brand **new** you inside and out. The saying we all know that goes, "You are what you eat" is absolutely true in every way because our body physically uses what we feed it to renew and rebuild itself. If we feed it processed foods and junk, our future bodies will be rebuilt weaker with a lower immune system, more aches and pain, weaker hair and nails etc. But if we feed it lots of yummy nutritious fresh food high in vitamins and minerals, our future body will be healthy, full of energy, stronger and be able to fight off sickness and disease more effectively. This is why your long-term lifestyle and diet is so important. What sort of cells do you want to grow in the future? Unhealthy, damaged cells, lacking in nutrients and prone to sickness and disease or strong, healthy, vibrant cells because you are eating amazing nutritious foods?

Your body is like a blank Word document. **You** input what you want to say and print it off. Once it is printed, you cannot rub out the ink on the paper. You could white it out, but let's face it you will always notice the mark as a reminder of the mistake. The only way to make a correction is to go back into the document on your computer, make the edits or corrections and print it off again. This is essentially what we are doing when we detox correctly.

When you detox properly under supervision from a Nutritional Coach, you can achieve all of the following benefits.

- Eliminate as many toxic ingredients as possible to give the body a break and a clear out.
- Flood the body with nutrient dense foods, which start to rebuild brand new healthier cells all over your body.
- Create long-term good habits while getting rid of the old bad habits.

- Reset your taste buds so you don't like the taste of junk processed foods as much.
- Reduce and/or eliminate junk food and sugar cravings.
- Oh yes, excess fat cells will begin to melt away almost effortlessly as you flush away that toxic overload! HURRAY!

Most importantly it is NOT about starving or not eating anything for long periods of time.

Not only this, but if you suffer from a chronic illness, a detox can really help give you a boost. We stumbled across the link between safe detoxing and chronic illness when we first tried it. Josh's Sickle Cell disorder meant he was always tired, always in pain, living on 10 medications a day and going into hospital up to 20 times a year. Fast forward to now, after learning how to detox safely without deprivation and totally revamping his lifestyle, he very rarely has to take his medication and isn't in hospital nearly as much as before. No, he isn't perfect, but his life has changed almost unrecognisably from what it was previously. We have had a few clients who have come to us for weightloss, but as a side effect of following our programme have also massively improved their Crohn's disease and Irritable Bowel Syndrome symptoms. I am not saying we can heal everything and you must always get your doctor's advice before making dietary changes if you have a chronic illness, but you now know that by detoxing your body without depriving yourself, it is possible to change your life in more ways than simply weightloss.

CHAPTER 7:

The Nutrition PA's 6 Step Success Formula

Throughout this book, I have revealed the **TRUTH** that you need to know for you to lose weight the healthy way and keep it off too. You now have a 6 Step Success Formula.

1. Have a clear and defined goal, which is measured fairly.
2. Get your mindset in check. Be honest with yourself but don't beat yourself up. You are human after all. Emotional eating can be harder to beat than you think, so give yourself time.
3. Get educated in how your body works and about nutrition from a nutrition professional. Learn how to read your labels and understand what you are putting in your body. Remember low calorie or low fat does not always mean healthy.
4. Accountability and support is key, most people struggle on their own.
5. Get some fitness education from a fitness professional. They can show you what you need to do to sculpt that body!
6. Detox without deprivation – under the supervision of a nutritional professional where possible. Start your new lifestyle on a fresh clean slate.

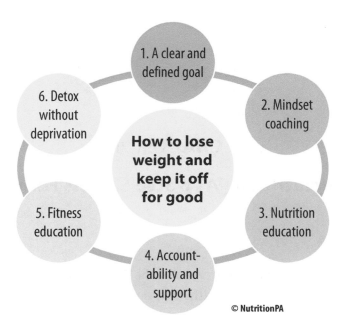

© NutritionPA

You have what it takes within you to achieve success, but you must stop seeing weightloss as a diet battle, where you lose some then you gain some. True weightloss is achievable without the long-term struggles and it doesn't need to feel like you are fighting a losing battle. I have seen this repetitively and on average, clients on our programme will lose a dress size in a month without breaking out a sweat and then keep going from success to success.

The journey is not easy, but wouldn't it be easier to do it only **once** and do it **right** rather than doing it again and again for the rest of your life? Seriously, the prospect of dieting for the rest of my life fills me with fear and despair to be frank. I could not think of anything worse. I always feel a sense of duty when I scroll my social media and see the collective cry of women struggling with their weightloss and paying a lot of money for the pleasure to do so. That is why I wrote this book.

Enough is enough, forget everything else you have tried before, remember it isn't you, it's them!

You can have success by:

- following the simple truths in this book;
- without dieting;
- by forgetting all the rubbish you have been told before about eating less food; and
- without starving yourself or setting foot in a gym!

Follow the 6 Step Success Formula.

However, I will say this, most people cannot do this alone. After many years of dieting and being bombarded with bad advice and junk food adverts, this is not easy to do alone. This isn't a criticism. It is a fact. Most successful people have a coach to help guide them and keep them on track. You don't get extra brownie points by saying; "I can do this on my own". You get the brownie points – and the brownie – by asking for help. The journey can be made much smoother if you accept help when it is offered to you. This can be a hard step. I have offered help to many people who have openly said they are struggling and do you know what they say to me? "Thanks, but no thanks." They are going to try this diet or that diet or this shake or that patch and those other pills. Always hoping that the next faddy thing is going to work all the while spending more and more money and ruining their metabolism and feeling fed up about the whole thing. My advice is stop hoping and start doing the things that are actually going to work, for real this time. I had a conversation with a lady once who told me she worked out 5 days a week and ate 2 meals a day, but wasn't losing any weight after 3 months. I asked if she was happy and she said; "No!" I offered help and she politely declined and said her Personal Trainer had given her instructions. Firstly, no offence, but if what she was doing was going to work it would have been working by now or at least started to work. Definition of insanity is doing the same thing again and again yet expecting different results. Not seeing any results across a prolonged period of time is a massive clue that what you are doing isn't working for you. Success leaves clues and so do failures. In other words, if you feel like you are getting success that is a clue it is working. However, if you feel frustrated, fed up, confused and hungry then they are clues that whatever it is you are doing, simply isn't working. Secondly, if you aren't happy doing what you are doing, stop doing it! Losing weight shouldn't make you unhappy and deflated. The journey should be empowering and invigorating. Every single one of our clients have said how empowered they feel once they have finished working with us. Who decided losing weight should be upsetting and not enjoyable? Why do we believe it needs to be hard work? No it won't always be easy, but it really needn't be soul destroying either. Remember that the longer you spend hoping that another missed meal will be the answer or hoping that a few more salad dinners will get you into those jeans, the harder it is going to be in the long run to finally lose weight. Dieting can mess up your metabolism LONG TERM. Your body won't know whether it is coming or going half the time and you can completely mess up its ability to work effectively and efficiently. This means that if you decide to make a real change and give up dieting for good, 3 years from now it will be twice as hard than if you decided to make that change **today**. We cannot go back in time. What is done is done. Let the past be the past. But you are fully in control of your future and only **you** can make a decision today never to diet again.

If you want to reach your goal for real this time, maybe it is time to have a chat with someone to help support you and remember it is 100% okay to have help. In fact, you will feel better once you have help to guide you and cheer you on. Why say, "No" to having your own little cheerleader? Not in the form of a diet club or a group of other women trying to 'figure it out' which is basically the blind leading the blind. I was a member of a group like that, a bunch of amazing women trying to lose weight together, offering advice and sharing successes. While this is great for moral support and motivation in some ways, in other ways this can totally ruin your chance of success. The diet that worked for her might not work for you. In fact, it could be dangerous for you. While that single lady can cook fresh food every day. You on the other hand, might not have the time as a married mum with 4 children and when you try her way, you end up feeling like a failure. The diet club leader or protein shake sales person isn't trained in nutrition or how the body works, they are trained in how to sell their products which again, may or may not work for you and doesn't take into consideration **you**, **your** body or **your** habits.

Who you can get help from is an important decision. You wouldn't ask your granny to fix your broken down car would you? No, you would ask a mechanic. Why would you ask an untrained person how you can lose weight the healthy way and keep it off? There are many, many health professionals who are weighting – get it? – for you to reach out. Shop around. Get a free session and see if your values match theirs and if you get along with them. If you feel you can talk to them. Finding the right person will make it easier for you to open up and move forward. Of course, I would recommend myself (obviously), but I might not be right for you. If I am what you need, great! But if not, I can point you in the direction of someone who is better suited to your individual needs. I have a huge network of amazing nutrition professionals who specialise in all sorts of different areas and I am always happy to make a referral if needs be.

Now I know some people will say, "nutrition coaching costs too much money". Well, it doesn't have to cost the earth. Shop around. A good coach shouldn't need you to stay with them forever. You might only need a few sessions with a nutritional therapist to get you kickstarted. If you have had a gym membership that you did or didn't use, then you can afford a Health Coach. Aside from that, you have to ask yourself; "Would you put a price on your health?" Josh and I used to fight about this all the time. When he was on his journey trying to be free from his Sickle Cell pain, he started spending a lot of money and I got upset because I didn't want to spend so much money. It was more money than we could afford. Coaching, herbal medicines, juicers, blenders, organic food, supplements, water distiller...the list went on but let's just say we maxed out more than one credit card along the way. Now, I am not suggesting you do this, not at all. Josh's health was deteriorating very badly and this was something he had to do to get a better quality of life. But what I am saying is to ask yourself, "How much is your health worth to you?" Can you cut back on something for a month or two for you to get the proper support you want? Most people find when they switch off Cable, stop buying takeaways or make their own morning coffee rather than getting it from Starbucks, they can free up some cash to use elsewhere. What you do is up to you. But make sure you stop and think about it so you know you are making a fully informed decision about your next step. Have look at your options. See how much it would really cost. Send me an email and I will see if I can connect you with someone. Whatever you do, please don't finish this book and put it down to collect dust or to take up space on your phone or tablet memory.

The most important thing you can do now is you make a decision; a decision to take on board the points in this book; a decision to stop listening to all the rubbish about low fat diet foods; a decision to make that change and make it for good this time. You don't have to do it all at once. This can be overwhelming. It is better to do it one step at a time, little by little. Each time you successfully make a change no matter how small, remember to reward yourself. (Not with food remember, we aren't dogs). Go to the spa, book a weekend getaway, have your nails done, go to the movies or take a bubble bath. Reward yourself for all 'those little wins' and all those barriers you overcame. In fact, you can reward yourself for reaching the end of this book! It is not easy learning new things and I have thrown a lot of new information at you. I have challenged you to rewire your thinking and start from scratch. That can be hard work and you deserve a little reward for that. For being open-minded enough to look into a new and exciting way to move forward. Feel happy you took a step and give yourself more than a pat on the back. What good is a pat on the back, anyway? A pat doesn't make me feel any better, but a massage on the back? Now we are talking!

As a bonus and to get you kickstarted, I have enlisted Josh to help me with some recipes to show you that eating healthier needn't be a bore or a chore. We have chocolate goodies, we have biscuits, and we have all sorts of yummy, scrummy foods to get your juices flowing. And to prove how fun detoxing our way is, these are all fully detox approved on our programme! There are some really simple and basic swaps that you can make while experimenting in the kitchen. Swap wheat pasta for spelt pasta, swap regular sugar for coconut sugar, or swap dairy for coconut or almond alternatives. It is not about giving up the foods we love; it is about finding the healthier alternatives. It's a little game I love to play with our clients. They tell me what guilty pleasure they are craving and we source a healthier version for them to enjoy, guilt free!

Have fun with it and enjoy getting back in the kitchen. More importantly start enjoying your food again.

Today is the day you make a U turn. Today is the day you make a change. Today is the day your life can change.

Today is the day you deserve success!

CHAPTER 8:

Healthy Recipes

Kickstart your healthy eating with the following recipes from me, with help from my lovely chef, Josh.

Let's start with SMOOTHIES! This is my favourite subject because breakfast is and always will be the most important meal of the day and a smoothie can be a perfect breakfast. Your breakfast sets the tone for the rest of the day. It either encourages bingeing and junk food cravings or it helps guide you and keeps you focussed and full of energy. This is why almost every morning you will find us drinking smoothies together in the kitchen as a family. Or if I am in a rush, I pour it into my shaker cup and take it to go. Actually in reality, the latter is far more realistic these days because I love my sleep too much and I usually run out of time to sit leisurely in the morning.

As we know, not all smoothies are made the same. We want to make a breakfast that is quick and easy while being nutritious and FILLING! That's the key word here...filling!

A good blender is an essential part of making deliciously smooth shakes that are filling and nutritious. My personal recommendations are a Vitamix or Nutribullet. You can also use a hand blender if on a budget and I have a friend who uses her food processor, but bear in mind that small seeds like hemp seeds will not blend as well with a hand blender or food processor.

How to build a PERFECT, healthy, nutritious, weightloss boosting breakfast smoothie!

STEP ONE – Choose your GREENS

Greens are key to your smoothies because they will help alkalise and detox your body and aid your weightloss. They are FULL of vital nutrients. A great way to get calcium, great for energy, great for detoxing, great for burning fat, great for you heart, great for the gut. Greens are the key to vitality and are often overlooked. It is tricky to eat a lot of greens, especially if you don't like them like me, but by putting them in your morning smoothie each day will give you great benefits.

The popular choices are either kale or spinach. Or for a more subtle flavour, we recommend spinach. We start clients off on 1 or 2 cups as you get used to the taste, but as you go on you can add more and more. I tend to have around 3 cups and Josh? Well, he adds the whole bag! LOL! I stick to spinach as I am a creature of habit but josh will try all sorts of greens. He will have kale, watercress (if you are brave with tastes!), coriander, parlane, parsley and even dandelion which he got from the garden! You can buy it but we were chuffed to find that it grows wild like a weed!

STEP TWO – Choose your FRUIT

As well as being full of nutrients, fruit adds a tasty flavour that will disguise the tastes of the greens and keep you fuller for longer. Hurray! The best choice for weightloss is berries. If you feel like it isn't filling enough, add an extra banana! But remember, fruit is good so feel free to experiment with your flavours.

STEP THREE – Choose your FATS

Yes, we said FATS! Good fats are good for weightloss. Good fats actually help you BURN bad fat in your body; so get stuck in! Popular choices are a handful of almonds, a tablespoon of flax seeds, hemp seeds, pine nuts, walnuts or almond butter.

STEP FOUR – Choose Your LIQUID

Choose either water, coconut water, or a non-dairy milk such as hemp, coconut milk or almond milk. The best brands of milk we have found are KOKO for coconut milk, or yogurt and Almond Breeze for almond milk. We also sometimes use half milk and half water. It saves money and spreads the milk further.

STEP FIVE – Choose your PROTEIN POWDER (optional)

We highly recommend a plant based protein powder. Free of artificial flavours, colours, sugars, sweeteners, diary, soy, whey and gluten. The best brands we have found are Sunwarrior and Arbonne which both do a variety of flavours as well as a flavour-free alternative too.

Smoothie Ideas

Top tips

- For added thickness or to feel fuller for longer, add a teaspoon or two of chia seeds. Chia seeds absorb water and expand in your tummy to give you that full feeling. But remember, as they are soaking up your water to fill your tummy, you need to make sure you re-hydrate to compensate for this. It is beneficial to soak your seeds for 10 to 15 minutes beforehand too.
- If you are adding nuts for optimal digestion, we advise to soak them overnight before you use them.
- Use frozen fruit or ice to make sure your smoothies are cool. There's nothing worse than a warm smoothie.
- With all the recipes you can edit quantities to suit your taste.

- Use organic ingredients wherever possible to minimise the toxins. You will be surprised to find plenty of organic farmers at the market with decent prices and even in Asda they have a large range of organic at good prices
- Remember your goal is to UP those dark leaf greens gradually.

Pina Banana Colada

- **2 scoops plain protein powder**
- **1 – 2 bananas, depending on size**
- **1 – 2 cups pineapple chunks**
- **1 cup of greens, spinach or kale**
- **1 cup coconut chunks**
- **1 teaspoon hemp seeds**

coconut milk to desired thickness

add ice and blend

Purple Power

- **1 – 2 scoops of vanilla protein powder**
- **1 cup of greens, spinach or kale**
- **1 cup of frozen mixed berries**
- **1 teaspoon of ground flax seeds**

water to desired thickness

add ice and blend

Almond Choca Lotta

- **2 scoops chocolate protein powder or raw cacao**
- **1 cup of greens, spinach or kale**
- **1 banana**
- **1 – 2 teaspoons of almond butter**
- **1 teaspoon hemp seeds**

coconut milk to desired thickness

cinnamon and nutmeg to taste

add ice and blend

Jamaican Ginger Bread

- 2 scoops chocolate protein powder or raw cacao
- 1 cup of greens, spinach or kale
- 1 banana
- 1 teaspoon flax seeds or hemp seeds
- 1 teaspoon chia seeds
- ¼ teaspoon each of nutmeg, cinnamon and ginger, or for an extra kick, add real ginger chunks!

water to desired thickness

add ice and blend

Green Power!

- 3 – 4 cups of greens, spinach or kale
- 10 – 15 dates
- 1 – 2 bananas, depending on the taste you want
- 2 teaspoons of hemp seeds

water to desired thickness

add ice and blend

Refresher

- ½ cucumber
- 1 cup of greens, spinach or kale
- 2 apples
- 3 pears
- 1 cup of mango pieces
- 1 tablespoon goji berries
- 7 dates

water to desired thickness

add ice and blend

Green Strawberries 'n Cream

- 10 strawberries
- 2 – 3 cups of spinach

- **2 – tablespoons of dairy free coconut yogurt**
- **1 teaspoon hemp seeds**

coconut milk to desired thickness

add ice and blend

Chocolate Orange

- **2 scoops chocolate protein or raw cacao**
- **2 oranges, peeled**
- **1 small banana**
- **1 – 2 cups spinach**
- **1 pinch of cinnamon**
- **1 pinch of ginger powder or a small piece of real ginger**

coconut milk for desired thickness

add ice and blend

Tutti Frutti

- **mixture of greens, kale, parsley, romaine lettuce...**
- **2 bananas**
- **2 apples**
- **2 pears**
- **6 strawberries**
- **handful of blueberries**
- **1 teaspoon hemp seeds**

water to desired thickness

add ice and blend

Strawberry Cheesecake

- **1 cup greens, spinach or kale**
- **1 scoop vanilla protein powder**
- **3 cups strawberries**
- **1 teaspoon cinnamon,**
- **1 cup dairy free soy free coconut yogurt**

coconut milk to desired thickness

add ice and blend

Food Ideas

Top tips

- Buy organic where possible to reduce toxins. We all assume organic is too expensive, but next time you are in your supermarket have a look and you will be surprised what you can get. Organic spinach, broccoli, onions, garlic and mushrooms for example, can be bought without breaking the bank.
- Use cartons of pulses/tomatoes rather than cans. The aluminium cans are toxic to the body. Tesco and Sainsbury's sell cartons and they are organic too!
- Recipes with 1 asterisk (*) can be made in bulk and put in the fridge for 2 or 3 days.
- Recipes with 2 asterisks (**) can be made in bulk and put in the freezer for 2 or 3 days.
- To make the prep time quicker, we use a food processor to chop onions, garlic, bell peppers or anything else that requires chopping. This really speeds up the process.
- The only salt we use is pink Himalayan salt because it is much better for us than table salt...plus it's pink! What more do you want?
- These recipes are made specifically to our tastes. Once you have tried it once to see how it is, feel free to experiment for your own tastes and preferences.
- As much as Josh and I love cooking and are great at creating our own nutritious meals, we aren't professional chefs! Quantities may be a teeeensy little bit off in places, but again, go with the flow and experiment to your own taste. We believe cooking should be about having fun and getting creative, so go for it!

Frittata

INGREDIENTS

- **2 tablespoons coconut oil**
- **½ medium red onion, finely sliced**
- **1 cup sliced mushrooms**
- **½ courgette, diced**
- **100g spinach**
- **½ red pepper, sliced**
- **6 olives, chopped (optional)**

- a handful sundried tomatoes, chopped
- 5 very large organic eggs
- 2 tablespoons coconut flour
- 1 teaspoon (aluminium free) baking powder
- ¼ cup almond milk
- 6 plum tomatoes, halved
- Himalayan salt and paprika

METHOD

1. Heat 1 tablespoon of oil in a pan and sauté the onions until lightly browned.
2. Add the garlic, mushrooms, courgette and peppers and season with paprika and salt. Continue to heat until cooked and set to one side.
3. In a bowl mix together the eggs, coconut flour, baking powder and almond milk.
4. Add the cooked vegetable mix to the egg mixture.
5. Add in the sundried tomatoes and olives.
6. Grease a pan with the remainder of the oil (it needs to be able to go in the oven). Pour the mixture into the pan and place the halved tomatoes on top. Place on the heat for 5 minutes until the mix starts to set slightly.
7. Place in the oven at 180°C (fan assisted oven) until it is firm and cooked through.
8. Turn out onto a plate and cut into slices.

Top Tip

To stop sticking, grease the pan with coconut oil and line the bottom of the pan with baking paper. Grease the baking paper with coconut oil and pour the mixture on top. It helps to turn the frittata out.

Creatan Style Baked Butter Beans*

INGREDIENTS

- 5 cartons/cans butter beans
- 1 red onion
- 1 garlic clove
- 3 sticks of celery
- 2 cans of chopped tomato

- 2 fresh tomatoes
- 2 teaspoons coconut sugar
- 1 large bay leaf (or 2 small)
- Himalayan salt to taste

METHOD

1. Heat a small amount of coconut oil in a pan and fry the finely chopped onion and garlic until soft.
2. Add in the celery, tomatoes, sugar, bay leaf and 1 cup of water and bring to the boil. Simmer for 15 – 20 minutes.
3. Add in the butter beans and stir until coated in the tomato mixture.
4. Transfer everything to an ovenproof dish and bake at 200°C for about 40 minutes, turning occasionally to ensure even cooking.
5. Serve as a side dish or on its own.

Ahisha's Curry (which is the absolute best!)**

INGREDIENTS

- coconut oil for frying
- 2 small red onions or 1 large red onion
- 1 garlic clove
- 1 ½ tablespoons mild curry powder
- 2 ¼ teaspoons pink Himalayan salt
- 1 teaspoon mix herbs
- 1 teaspoon basil
- 1 teaspoon paprika
- 2 bay leaves
- cayenne powder to taste
- 100 – 200 grams creamed coconut (the one in the block usually found in the Indian or Caribbean section of the supermarket)
- 6 cartons (cans) organic chickpeas
- 3 cartons (cans) organic chopped tomato

METHOD

1. Finely chop the onions and garlic. I blitz mine in the food processor for ease and speed.
2. Heat a small amount of coconut oil in a pan.
3. Add the chopped garlic, onion, curry powder, salt and cook until onions are soft and stir well, about 5 – 10 minutes.
4. Add in the drained chickpeas and season with the mixed herbs, paprika and mix together thoroughly and cook for 10 minutes.
5. Add the chopped tomato, basil, bay leaves and cayenne pepper to taste (my preference is 6 'shakes') and mix thoroughly.
6. Add in 100 – 200 grams of creamed coconut. The more you add, the creamier the curry. Make sure it is melted by stirring through.
7. Once coconut cream has all melted and mixed in, simmer and cover for 5 – 10 minutes, stirring occasionally to prevent sticking. If you find it is too thick add small amounts of water.

Top Tip

If you find you have added too much cayenne, add more coconut cream to make it milder again.

Serve with quinoa and avocado.

Quinoa Pizza Base (makes 2 small pizza bases)

INGREDIENTS

- **1 cup quinoa**
- **juice 1 lemon or lime**
- **1 teaspoon ground turmeric (optional)**
- **Himalayan salt to taste**

METHOD

1. Soak the quinoa overnight or for at least 4 hours in cold water.
2. When you are ready to make your bases simply rinse and drain the quinoa in a sieve. Put it in the food processor, add the lemon juice and seasoning and blitz for around 5 – 7 minutes until it looks like paste.

3. Pour the mixture out on a baking sheet. I put a tiny drop of coconut oil on the baking sheet for greasing, so the base doesn't stick to the sheet, spread it thinly and put in the oven at 180°C for around 10 – 12 minutes, until it's turning slightly golden).

4. Take it out of the oven, put the sauce – tomato paste or pesto works really well – and your chosen toppings and place it back in the oven for another 5 – 7 minutes, until it's turning slightly brown.

Top Tip

You don't need to top it with cheese, be creative!

Simple Pasta

INGREDIENTS

- **spelt pasta (enough for 2 to 3 servings)**
- **1 – 2 chopped avocados**
- **5 – 10 chopped plum tomatoes**
- **Himalayan salt to taste**
- **cayenne pepper to taste**
- **extra virgin cold pressed olive oil**

METHOD

1. Cook the pasta as stated on the packet.
2. Chop tomatoes and avocado and combine in a bowl with a few drops of olive oil. Stir well until the avocado starts to break down a little, to create a creamy texture.
3. Combine with slightly cooled pasta, add salt to taste and eat!

Top Tip

Wheat pasta can create bloating and gut irritations. It can be replaced by spelt, lentil, pea or kumut pasta. There are many other types of pasta available these days so go and check them out.

Butternut Squash Soup*

This is an easy to prepare, delicious healthy soup, which everyone will love! Feel free to play around with vegetables you like. This recipe is a basic guide to create a hearty, warming soup.

INGREDIENTS

- ½ to 1 whole butternut squash, diced, about 1 ½ cups, use more or less depending on your taste
- 2 sweet potatoes, diced
- sesame oil to fry
- small red onion, diced
- ½ red bell pepper, diced
- 1 clove garlic, chopped
- 32 ounces of salt free and gluten free vegetable stock/broth OR use half vegetable stock and half water, about 425 grams (15 ounces) each
- 2 teaspoons fresh chopped rosemary or more to taste, use dried if you don't have fresh available
- 2 teaspoons fresh chopped thyme or more to taste, use dried if you don't have fresh available
- 1 tablespoon dried basil
- ½ teaspoon Himalayan salt or more or less, to your taste

METHOD

1. Heat the sesame oil in a large, heavy bottomed soup pan on medium heat.
2. Add onion, garlic, red pepper and sauté until translucent.
3. Add all the vegetables, seasonings and veggie stock.
4. Bring to a gentle boil and lower to a simmer.
5. Cook until all the vegetables are tender, but not mushy.
6. Stir occasionally, for about 30 minutes.
7. Add a little water if needed.

Red Pepper, Tomato and Lentil Soup*

INGREDIENTS

- 3 cartons (cans) of lentils
- 1 carton (can) chopped tomato
- 1 to 2 red pepper
- 1 medium onion
- 1 large garlic clove
- 1 ½ teaspoon coconut vinegar
- ¼ teaspoon chipotle flakes (add more if you want a spicier soup)
- 1 teaspoon smoked paprika
- 1 teaspoon mixed herbs
- ¼ teaspoon cumin
- 1 teaspoon coconut sugar
- 1 teaspoon Himalayan salt

METHOD

1. Finely chop the garlic and onions and fry in a little coconut oil until soft.
2. Finely chop red pepper and add to the pot.
3. Add the cumin, ½ teaspoon paprika and ½ teaspoon mixed herbs and combine well.
4. Add the chopped tomato, chipotle flakes, coconut vinegar, coconut sugar and ½ teaspoon salt, mix well.
5. Stir in the lentils with the rest of the of the salt, paprika and mixed herbs, which should be ½ teaspoon of each, staggering the seasoning in this way adds a real depth to the end flavour.
6. Blend the entire mixture in a food processor until desired consistency. Once blended, pour back into your pot gently simmer for 5 minutes. Add water to desired thickness, I usually add a mug of water.

Super Salad!

INGREDIENTS

- 4 – 6 cups fresh salad greens, such as lettuce, red-leaf lettuce, spinach or romaine, mix it up!

- 1 small to medium handful rocket/arugula or kale
- ½ avocado peeled and diced, or use the whole avocado if you like
- 1 – 2 or more tomatoes, diced or a handful chopped cherry tomatoes
- ½ medium cucumber, chopped into bite size pieces
- 3 – 4 chopped fresh basil sprigs
- 4 – 5 chopped fresh coriander sprigs
- 2 tablespoons toasted pine nuts or almonds, spread on a baking sheet and roast at 300°C for a few minutes, they toast fast so keep an eye on them or add them raw.

METHOD

1. Choose a big salad bowl with lots of room.
2. Add the lettuce, rocket/arugula, kale, avocado, tomato and cucumber and whatever other veggies you're playing with. Top with the dandelion greens and herbs. Sprinkle with the seeds and nuts. Lightly salt and pepper if you like.
3. Drizzle with dressing (ideas below), directly onto the salad and toss and voila! Your super salad is ready for you.

Dressing Ideas

- **Citrus Dressing**
- **2 ½ tablespoons extra-virgin olive oil**
- **1 ½ tablespoons coconut vinegar**
- **Juice of ½ lemon**
- **Juice of ½ lime**
- **Whisk together until creamy**

Avocado Dressing

- 1 large ripe avocado
- 1 garlic clove
- ¼ teaspoon chipotle pepper flakes (optional)
- 2 tablespoon lime juice
- 2 teaspoon extra virgin olive oil
- ½ cup water

Blend all ingredients together and enjoy!

Quinoa Tabbouleh Salad*

INGREDIENTS

- 170 grams quinoa
- 1 tablespoon olive oil
- 4 tablespoons lemon juice
- ½ teaspoon Himalyan salt
- 3 tomatoes, diced
- 1 cucumber, diced
- 1 bunch of spring onions, chopped
- 60 grams fresh parsley, chopped
- 1 avocado (optional) if making in bulk, make sure to add the avocado fresh each time

METHOD

1. Cook quinoa according to packet instructions and cool to room temperature; fluff with a fork.
2. Meanwhile in a large bowl, combine olive oil, salt, lemon juice, tomatoes, cucumber, spring onions and parsley.
3. Stir in cooled quinoa.

Flaxseed crackers*

INGREDIENTS

- 200 grams ground flaxseeds
- juice from ½ lemon
- 1 crushed garlic cloves
- 1 teaspoon fresh ginger
- 1 handful fresh herbs
- salt and pepper
- olive oil to blend

METHOD

1. Blend all ingredients until combined.
2. Spread on a baking paper until ¼ inch thick or less.
3. Place in oven at 50°C or fan assisted oven 30°C or gas mark ¼.
4. Turn over after 6 – 8 hours. Dehydration takes around 12 hours. The longer you leave them, the crispier they will be!

Kale Chips

INGREDIENTS

- **large head of kale**
- **small bowl of olive oil**
- **pink Himalayan salt**

METHOD

1. Preheat oven to 220°C or 200°C fan assisted oven or gas mark 7.
2. Remove kale from stalk, cutting greens into strips.
3. Place a little olive oil in bowl, dip your fingers in and rub a light coating over the kale.
4. Lay the kale on a baking sheet and bake for 5 minutes or until it starts to turn a little brown.
5. Turn the kale over, add a little salt or curry or cumin to taste and bake for another 5 minutes.

The World's Easiest Biscuits (Makes about 16 biscuits)

INGREDIENTS

- **2 cups finely ground almond flour (227 grams)**
- **½ teaspoon baking powder**
- **⅓ cup dark date syrup or honey (100 grams)**
- **2 teaspoons vanilla extract**

METHOD

1. Adjust an oven rack to the middle position and heat the oven to 176°C. Line a rimmed baking sheet with baking paper.
2. Whisk the almond flour and baking powder together in a medium bowl. Switch to a wooden spoon and stir in the maple syrup and vanilla. Stir until a sticky dough forms and holds together.
3. Drop rounded tablespoons of the dough onto the prepared baking sheet, about one inch apart. For crisp biscuits, press down the dough lightly with the flat bottom of a drinking glass or measuring cup. If the glass sticks to the dough, dip the bottom in water. For softer biscuits, don't press down the dough so much.
4. Bake until the edges are golden brown, about 12 minutes. Allow the cookies to cool on the pan for about 3 minutes and transfer to a wire rack to cool completely. Cool baking sheet between batches.

Protein Brownie Bars

INGREDIENTS

- **½ cup almond milk**
- **½ cup of medjool dates or prunes**
- **½ cup chocolate protein powder**
- **¼ cup raw cacao powder**
- **¼ cup coconut flour**
- **½ cup egg whites or aquafaba (the juice in a can of chick peas)**
- **¾ teaspoon baking powder**

Mix – Pour – Bake – Enjoy!

Bake for 35 minutes on 160C.

Tahini Choc Cacao Cookies

INGREDIENTS

- **1 can of chickpeas, rinsed**
- **1 scoop chocolate protein powder or raw cacao**
- **½ cup of tahini, unhulled**
- **¼ cup almond butter**
- **1 teaspoon baking powder**

- pinch of pink Himalayan salt
- handful cacao nibs

METHOD

1. Preheat your oven to 175°C and line a baking tray with baking paper.
2. Combine all ingredients excluding cacao nibs in a food processor, until it looks like cookie dough.
3. Add in cacao nibs.
4. Roll dough into balls and flatten into biscuits. Wet your hands to prevent sticking.
5. Bake for approximately 12 minutes, until golden. They should stay soft and dense like a brownie.

*Mango Chia Pudding **

INGREDIENTS

- ¼ cup chia seeds
- ¾ cup coconut milk
- ¼ cup coconut cream
- 1 teaspoon vanilla extract
- 1 mango
- 1 teaspoon honey or date syrup
- shredded coconut (optional)

METHOD

1. Mix all the ingredients until they are combined well, cover and keep in the fridge overnight or for a minimum of 6 hours.
2. Top with mango and organic shredded coconut, or alternatively, place everything in the blender for a nice smooth consistency. You can also make this with any fruit that takes your fancy.

Chocolate Chia Pudding *

INGREDIENTS

- 1 ¼ cup to 1 ½ cup unsweetened almond milk or coconut, as needed to thin out
- ¼ cup chia seeds
- 1 teaspoon honey or date syrup
- ½ teaspoon raw cacao powder
- 1 teaspoon chocolate/protein (optional)
- Raw cacao nibs or strawberries for garnish (optional)

METHOD

1. In a large bowl, whisk together all of the ingredients, starting with the milk until the clumps are gone.
2. Place in the fridge for 1 – 2 hours, until thick or overnight.
3. Stir well, add more milk if desired to achieve thickness, and serve chilled.
4. Nice with mixed berries/cherries, which reminds me of chocolate gateau. As with the mango chia pudding, you can also blend everything together for a smoother consistency.

A FINAL WORD FOR YOU...

I have had an amazing time writing this book for you! My hope is that you can take a few nuggets of wisdom and start smashing through those blocks and finally start seeing the results you have been looking for.

As promised, if you wish to reach out for a chat on how to get started on your new journey feel free to email me on: *info@nutritionpa.com*

I am more than happy to give you a kickstart and get you going or point you in the right direction to someone who might be more suited to your specific needs.

At the very least, let this book be your new guide to self-empowerment and self-love. Take the pressure off and enjoy food again. Stop depriving yourself of the foods you love by giving yourself a cheat meal and gradually, little by little you can change your diet, your lifestyle and create something truly amazing! I look back at my past and I laugh at what I used to eat. I look in my fridge now and wonder whose house I am in and you know what? I feel so proud when I realise it's all me! I am certainly not perfect, but it's a new and improved me and I LOVE IT!

Now it's your turn. Let your dieting officially **stop** on Monday.

Happy eating 'yall!

REFERENCES AND FURTHER RESOURCES

1. Dr Kevin Hall, United States National Institutes for Health, www.nih.gov

2. Stan Reents, 2000, Sport and Exercise Pharmacology, www.amazon.co.uk/Sport-Exercise-Pharmacology-Stan-Reents/dp/0873229371

3. American College of Sports Medicine, Orlando, Florida, USA, www.amssm.org

4. Wayne Wescott PHD, South Shore YMCA Quincy, Massachusetts, http://ssymca.org/health-education-lifestyle-programs/

5. Gaynor Pengelly, 2014, *Cut the soaring cost of dieting down to size: Average woman spends £25,000 on weight plans in a lifetime – but getting trim needn't cost a fortune*, Financial Mail on Sunday, www.thisismoney.co.uk

6. Melissa Whitworth, 2008, Big Fat Lie, The Telegraph, www.telegraph.co.uk/lifestyle/wellbeing/diet/3353110/Big-fat-lie.html

7. P T Williams & P D Wood, 2006, *The effects of changing exercise levels on weight and age-related weight gain*, International Journal of Obesity, volume 30, www.ncbi.nlm.nih.gov/pubmed/16314878

ABOUT THE AUTHOR

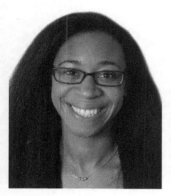

Photo credit c/o Sue Odell

Ahisha Ferguson is a Nutritional Therapist and Health Coach who started her adult life as a professional dancer and actor. She has performed on many stages from London's West End, to Disneyland Paris and the MGM Grand in Las Vegas. Her professional interest in heath began when she started caring for her husband Josh, who suffers from a chronic blood disorder. Ahisha went back to school to study nutrition and set up her business, 'Nutrition PA', to help people improve their health through food. In January 2017, Ahisha's mother and former Mayor of Stevenage, Sherma Batson MBE, suddenly passed away. While Ahisha dealt with her grief, she followed her dream of writing her first book, to help women lose weight and keep it off without dieting. Ahisha openly shares her knowledge of the diet industry, health and nutrition, as well as her personal experiences to help other women break free from dieting and finally achieve the success they deserve.

CONTACT

Email: info@nutritionpa.com

Website: www.nutritionpa.com

FB: www.facebook.com/nutritionpa/

FB: www.facebook.com/dietstopsmonday/

CPSIA information can be obtained
at www.ICGtesting.com
Printed in the USA
LVHW07s1702250218
567813LV00005B/11/P